Why is **Pumping Insulin** different? It's an insider's view, with the unique insights of a dedicated clinician and pump user, one who has the longest personal experience and who has trained more pumpers than any writer I know. From the broadest generalities to the most minute details (and secrets you will not find elsewhere), this book prepares you for success. It's easy to use, complete, and a pleasure to read.

The rapidly increasing popularity of insulin pumping is testament to its being the gold standard for best control with insulin. I hope this book encourages more people to realize the benefits of insulin pumping and helps those already using it to fine-tune their skills.

— Daniel Einhorn, MD, FACP, FACE
    Diabetes and Endocrine Associates
    Director, Sharp HealthCare Diabetes
    Associate Clinical Professor of Medicine, UCSD

"**Pumping Insulin** truly deserves the nickname of the insulin pumper's bible. It's the first book I recommend to people when they ask about trying to manage this disease. I even recommend it to folks who are not pumping (I read it a year prior to starting pump therapy). I firmly believe this book should be mandated reading for all medical professionals.

The information on blood glucose patterns is great It taught me that my blood glucose patterns were not unique, were not abnormal and were something that I could take control of. I didn't feel alone with my inconsistent results. The practical, simply stated advice is tremendous. I still return to this book whenever I find myself out in the weeds, wandering more than I want to."

— Bob Burnett
    Webmaster, Bob's Corner of the Web
    home.twcny.rr.com/bobscorner/

"I read **Pumping Insulin** before I began pump therapy. Because the information was so simple to understand it gave me the confidence to start on an infusion pump. Now, I regularly go back to **Pumping Insulin** when I have any questions or problems. The answers and instructions are always logical and easy to follow.

It is the best book on diabetes self-care that I own, with or without pump information. My recommendation to anyone thinking about pump therapy or getting ready to go on a pump ....GET THIS BOOK FIRST."

— Linda McClure
    Executive Director of International Diabetes Athletes Assoc. and pumper

Insulin pump companies in the U.S.:

Animas Corporation	(877) 937-7867	www.animascorp.com
Dana Diabcare USA	(866) 342-2322	www.theinsulinpump.com
Disetronic Medical Systems, Inc.	(800) 280-7801	www.disetronic-usa.com
Medtronic Minimed	(800) 646-4633	www.minimed.com
Smiths Medical MD, Inc	(800) 826-9703	www.CozMore.com

The latest pump information at our web site:

Current insulin pumps	www.diabetesnet.com/diabetes_technology/insulinpumps.php
Pump models & features	www.diabetesnet.com/diabetes_technology/insulin_pump_models.php
Infusions sets	www.diabetesnet.com/diabetes_technology/infusion_sets.php
Continuous monitors	www.diabetesnet.com/diabetes_technology/new_monitoring.php
The Insulin Wizard	www.diabetesnet.com/diabetes_tools/

Other web sites of interest in pumping or diabetes

Children With Diabetes	www.childrenwithdiabetes.com
Diabetes Health	www.diabeteshealth.com
Topix.net	www.topix.net/health/diabetes
American Diabetes Assoc.	www.diabetes.org
Insulin Pumpers Group	www.insulin-pumpers.org
Medline	www.ncbi.nlm.nih.gov/PubMed/
Clinical trials in diabetes	www.centerwatch.com/patient/studies/area4.html
Nutrition and carb data	www.medexplorer.com/nutrition/nutrition.dbm

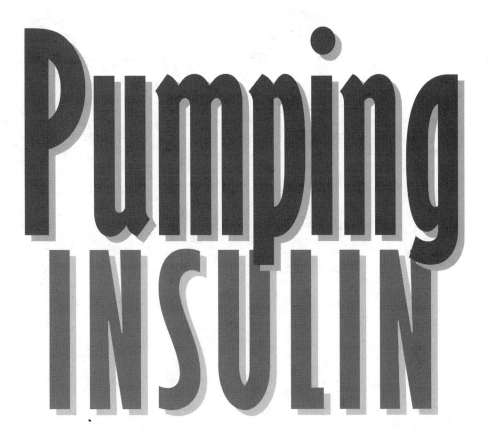

Pumping INSULIN

Everything You Need For Success With An Insulin Pump

by John Walsh, P.A., C.D.E., and Ruth Roberts, M.A.

Torrey Pines Press
San Diego

Torrey Pines Press
1030 West Upas Street
San Diego, California 92103-3821
1-619-497-0900

Library of Congress Cataloging in Publication Data

Walsh, John and Roberts, Ruth

Pumping Insulin:

Everything you need for success with an insulin pump, 3rd edition
by John Walsh, P.A., C.D.E. and Ruth Roberts, M.A.

p. cm.
Includes bibliographical references.
Includes index.
1. Diabetes Popular Books
2. Diabetes Insulin
3. Diabetes Insulin-dependent diabetes
4. Diabetes Research
5. Insulin Therapeutic use
I. Title

Library of Congress Card Number: 00-190817
ISBN 1-884804-84-5 $23.95 Paperback

Printed in the United States of America
10 9 8 7 6 5 4 3

More Praise...

"I'm keeping **Pumping Insulin** on my short shelf of reference books, and I suspect I'll be using it more than most of them. This one book makes life with diabetes so much simpler and better. In fact, you'll find answers to questions you haven't yet learned enough to ask!

Pumping Insulin explains how to make your pump do what you want it to do. You'll have at your fingertips methods to fix blood sugar problems and a short cut to all the tedious math involved. The authors have worked out precise tables for figuring boluses and basals, for determining the insulin needed to lower highs, and for knowing how many carbs to eat before exercising, along with covering other common problems.

It's amazing how much help these authors pack into a single volume. Using it is like having your own personal consultant and trainer every step of the way."

> — Helen Oswalt
> Type 1 for 14 years and pumper for 9 months
> Lay diabetes educator and support group leader

"Good, practical information on insulin pump therapy is hard to find. **Pumping Insulin** is the most comprehensive publication for people with diabetes considering and using an insulin pump. This book covers everything from determining the basal ratio and bolus rates to carbohydrate counting to insulin infusion sites and much more, and it all comes from your personal as well as professional experience with diabetes and pumping. **Pumping Insulin** deals with many of the daily situations that arise with pumping that can't be found in a diabetes textbook. I truly enjoyed reading this book!"

> — Steve V. Edelman, MD
> Assoc. Professor of Medicine, Univ. of Cal., San Diego School of Medicine
> Founder of *Taking Control of Your Diabetes*, a seminar series that promotes
>   education, motivation, and self-advocacy for people with diabetes
> Type 1 diabetes since age 15, and pumper

"Fourteen years ago when I was diagnosed with Type 1 diabetes, I read the 1st Edition of **Pumping Insulin**. At that time, it was extremely valuable in helping me balance my active lifestyle while maintaining good glucose control.

Now the 3rd Edition is chock full of up-to-date information pertaining to today's insulin pumps. Armed with the knowledge in this book, you can adjust your diabetes regimen to your or your patients' lifestyle. It should be on the bookshelf of anyone who wears a pump and those who treat them."

> — Joe Largay, PA-C, CDE
> Clinical Instructor, University of North Carolina Diabetes Care Center

John Walsh and Ruth Roberts have chronicled excellent control and insulin pump therapy for over ten years. The 1st edition of **Pumping Insulin** set the standard of care for pumps in 1989. This 3rd edition shows they are still the leaders in the field. **Pumping Insulin** is written from first-hand experience of wearing a pump for 18 years and from training hundreds of pumpers on how to better use theirs. No diabetes library is complete without this terrific resource!

— Scott King, Publisher
Diabetes Interview, the newsmagazine for the diabetes community since 1991

"**Pumping Insulin** is required reading in our practice. We find it essential for both potential and present pump patients. The third edition makes the definitive guide to pumping even better!"

— Timothy Bailey, MD, FACP
North County Endocrine, San Diego

"Oh Boy! A new **Pumping Insulin**! Whether I have a serious pump problem or a small concern, I have always been so blest to count on John Walsh and Ruth Roberts for their insight, concern, and advice that comes from hard-fought, first-hand experience in the trenches of life with diabetes."

— John Rodosevich
Founder, Editor: San Diego Insulin Pumpers, since 1982
IDDM 35 yrs, pumper 18 yrs, mechanical engineer since I was a little boy

"You've done it again! As with each of your books, you continue to update both pumpers and diabetes health care professionals on ways to apply the latest technologies to ourselves and our patients. The new charts for the use of Humalog are especially helpful and will make applying your techniques easy for the many pumpers using Humalog. This is truly a user-friendly book.

Thanks for your continued dedication to excellence in diabetes education. It has been a pleasure to help with the editing of **Pumping Insulin**---I always learn so much!

— JoAnne Scott, RN, CDE
diabetes educator and pump wearer

" This book is ideal for those who have decided to take back control of their blood sugars and life. A pump is clearly the most appropriate tool to normalize blood sugars. **Pumping Insulin** provides everthing necessary for the success of the person who has chosen a pump to improve their life today and their future. This book is magnificent, once again an opus!"

— Alan Marcus, MD, FACP
Associate Clinical Professor, U.S.C. School of Medicine
President, South Orange County Endocrinology

About the Authors

John Walsh, P.A., C.D.E., is a Physician Assistant and Diabetes Clinical Specialist who has worked for the last six years in a private endocrine clinic in Escondido, CA. He has provided clinical care to thousands of people with diabetes in a wide variety of clinical settings, including 10 years of care in the Endocrine Division of a large HMO in San Diego. He has worn a pump for 18 years, and started and followed over 400 people on pumps.

In addition, Mr. Walsh is a popular presenter on a wide variety of diabetes topics to physicians, health professionals and people with diabetes, including the American Diabetes Association, Juvenile Diabetes Foundation, International Diabetic Athletes Association, and hospital groups. He is on the Board of Directors for the International Diabetic Athletes Association and serves as President of Diabetes Services, Inc. He has authored or coauthored hundreds of diabetes articles, as well as diabetes books and booklets. He is a consultant for medical corporations and and has been a frequent guest on radio and TV programs as an authority on intensive diabetes management. His interests include identifying and providing clinical care for patients at risk of developing diabetes complications, stabilizing and reversing these complications, and enhancing blood sugar control through innovative methods.

Ruth Roberts, M.A., is CEO of The Diabetes Mall and a widely-read medical writer. She has also served as a corporate training administrator, technical writer, and instructional designer for fifteen years in San Diego. During the last 20 years, she has been involved in diabetes support groups, and has coauthored several books on diabetes. She is a professional member of the American Diabetes Association, on the Board of Directors for the International Diabetes Athletes Association, and the editor and frequent contributor to "Diabetes This Week", a weekly internet newsletter that is on the forefront of coverage of the latest developments in diabetes research and business. She has been a guest on "Living With Diabetes", and is an educational consultant on intensive self-management.

ALSO BY THE AUTHORS

Other books by John Walsh, P.A., C.D.E. and Ruth Roberts, M.A.:

STOP the Rollercoaster, *Torrey Pines Press, 1996*

Pocket Pancreas, *Torrey Pines Press, 1995, 1998*

Pumping Insulin, *second edition, Torrey Pines Press, 1994*

Insulin Pump Therapy Handbook, *1990*

Pumping Insulin, *first edition, 1989*

Diabetes Advanced Workbook, *1988*

Barb Schreiner, R.N., M.N., C.D.E. is a clinical nurse specialist and the associate director of the Diabetes and Endocrine Care Center at Texas Children's Hospital in Houston, TX. She is also an instructor for Baylor College of Medicine, Department of Pediatrics and serves on the adjunct faculty of the UT School of Nursing, Houston.

She has worked with individuals with diabetes for almost 25 years and is a Certified Diabetes Educator. Her volunteer work has included membership on the national Board of Directors of the American Diabetes Association, and chairman of the National Certification Board for Diabetes Educators.

She is a popular local, regional and national speaker and author on issues related to children with diabetes and serves as a consultant to many of the diabetes pharmaceutical companies. She is the recipient of numerous patient education awards and in 1997, Ms. Schreiner was honored as one of the 20 outstanding nurses in Houston.

Shannon I. Brow, R.N., B.S., C.D.E. is a pediatric diabetes nurse educator at Texas Children's Hospital in Houston. She is a Clinical Service Specialist for Disetronic and a certified pump trainer for MiniMed insulin pumps. Shannon has developed many patient education materials for use with children, their families, and adults in a variety of inpatient, outpatient, and clinic settings. She also teaches in local colleges of nursing.

Shannon has had diabetes since adolescence and began pumping in adulthood. She has jokingly been referred to as a "Peripatetic Diabetic," because of her love of travel. She "packs her diabetes in her suitcase" and travels around the world 1-2 times a year.

Shannon donates her summers as a medical staff volunteer to several day, weekend, and residential camping programs for children and young adults with diabetes. She is a member of the American Association of Diabetes Educators, and has served as an officer in the South Texas Association of Diabetes Educators. She is a volunteer for the American Diabetes Association and Juvenile Diabetes Foundation.

Acknowledgments

Pumping Insulin is the product of years of personal and professional experience with diabetes and insulin pumps. During this time, major contributions have been made by our patients, friends, family members, colleagues and fellow travelers.

Our heartfelt thanks go to the following individuals who graciously and critically reviewed and improved upon the third edition:

Helen Oswalt, support group leader and editor, par excellence, of San Diego, CA

Alan Marcus, M.D., Assoc. Clinical Professor of Medicine, U.S.C. School of Medicine, President of South Orange County Endocrinology of Laguna Hills, CA

Bob Burnett, pumper and webmaster of Bob's Corner of the Web home.twcny.rr.com/bobscorner/

John Rodosevich, Insulin Pumpers Support Group of San Diego, CA

Carol Wysham, M.D., of the Rockwood Clinic of Spokane, WA

Linda McClure, Executive Director of the International Diabetes Athletes Association in Phoenix, AZ

Timothy Bailey, M.D., F.A.C.P., North County Endocrine, Escondido, CA

Scott King, Publisher of *Diabetes Interview*, San Francisco, CA

JoAnne Scott, R.N., C.D.E. of Spokane, WA

Daniel Einhorn, M.D., F.A.C.P., F.A.C.E., Director of Sharp Healthcare Diabetes, Assoc. Clinical Professor of Medicine, U.C.S.D. School of Medicine, San Diego, CA

Steve V. Edelman, M.D., Founder of *Taking Control of Your Diabetes*, Assoc. Professor of Medicine, U.C.S.D School of Medicine, San Diego, CA

Joe Largay, P.A.C., C.D.E., Clinical Instructor, U.N.C. Diabetes Care Center of Raleigh, NC

Katie Odle of San Diego for editing, proofreading, and working on the index at short notice when we were close to our wit's end.

We and everyone with diabetes are indebted to:

The American Diabetes Association, the Juvenile Diabetes Foundation, the National Institiute of Health, and other national agencies that generously support diabetes education and research.

All the health practitioners and the 1,441 volunteers with diabetes who participated in the Diabetes Control and Complications Trial which confirmed what early pumpers and pump proponents already assumed—that controlling blood sugars makes people healthier and reduces the complications of diabetes.

We would also like to especially thank:

John Rodosevich for leadership in forming and maintaining the San Diego Pump Club over the last 18 years, and for writing with gentle wit and humor the *Insulin Pumpers Newsletter* which is widely read and enjoyed.

All the San Diego Pump Club Members and the thousands of pumpers who have made creating this book enjoyable and worthwhile.

All the reviewers of the first and second editions of **Pumping Insulin** who have contributed in their own special ways:

Marilyn James, management systems consultant of Del Mar, CA

Lois Jovanovic, M.D., Senior Scientist, Sansum Medical Clinic of Santa Barbara, CA

Sally Ann Drucker, Ph.D. of New York, NY

Jeffrey Hartman, M.D. of Spokane, WA

Laura Lyons, R.N., M.B.A of San Diego, CA

Don Leeds of Rancho Palos Verdes, CA

Irl B. Hirsch, M.D., and Ruth Farkas-Hirsch, M.S., R.N., C.D.E, University of Washington School of Medicine, Seattle, WA

Davida F. Kruger, R.N., M.S.N., C.D.E., Henry Ford Hospital

Charlene Freeman, R.N., C.D.E., McFarland Diabetes Center

Cover and chapter headings by Diane Steiner of Kanza Graphics, 2966 Kanza, Durham, KS 67438.

Table Of Contents

Tables

Workspaces

Other Graphics And Aids

Figures

Important Note

Pumping Insulin, 3rd Edition, has been developed as a guide to using insulin for diabetes control. Graphs, charts, examples, situations, and tips provide basic as well as advanced information related to the use of an insulin pump. Insulin requirements and treatment protocols differ significantly from one person to the next. The information included in this book should be used only as a guide. It is not a substitute for the sound medical advice of your personal physician or health care team.

Specific treatment plans, insulin dosages, and other aspects of health care for a person with diabetes, must be based on individualized treatment protocols under the guidance of your physician or health care team. The information in this book is provided to enhance your understanding of diabetes and insulin pumps so that you can manage the daily challenges you face. It can never be relied upon as a sole source for your personal diabetes regimen.

While every reasonable precaution has been taken in the preparation of this information, the authors and publishers assume no responsibility for errors or omissions, nor for the uses made of the materials contained herein and the decisions based on such use. No warranties are made, expressed, or implied, with regard to the contents of this work or to its applicability to specific individuals. The authors and publishers shall not be liable for direct, indirect, special, incidental, or consequential damages arising out of the use of or inability to use the contents of this book.

Read This!

Never use this book on your own! Any suggestion made in this book for improving blood sugar control with an insulin pump should only be followed with the approval and under the guidance of your personal physician. We have provided the best information and tools available to make your insulin pump do its job of normalizing your blood sugars.

However, this book is not enough. We have worked with pumpers who have used this information together with the guidance of their physician, and they have excelled. We have also seen pumpers who get themselves into trouble by a selective use of this or other material, and by ignoring or not seeking excellent medical advice.

Always seek the advice and guidance of your physician and health care team. No book can ever help you as much as they will. They have the benefit of objectivity and experience gained from working with many other pumpers. Your own participation in the process of good control is essential, but never minimize the importance of good professional advice and support. Teams win where individuals fail, and teamwork takes trust and communication from everyone.

We wish all users of this book good health and great control with their pumps.

Pump-Related Terms

BASAL INSULIN OR RATE

A continuous 24-hour delivery of insulin that matches background insulin need. When the basal is correctly set, the blood sugar does not rise or fall during periods in which the pump user is not eating. Basal rates are given as units/hour with typical rates between 0.4 u/hr and 1.6 u/hr.

CARB BOLUS

A spurt of insulin delivered quickly to match carbohydrates in an upcoming meal or snack. Most pumpers use between 1unit of Humalog for each 5 grams of carbohydrate and 1unit of Humalog for each 25 grams.

CATHETER

The plastic tube through which insulin is delivered between the pump and the insertion set.

HIGH BLOOD SUGAR BOLUS

A spurt of insulin delivered quickly to bring a high blood sugar back to normal. For most pumpers, one unit will lower the blood sugar between 20 and 100 mg/dl or points (between 1 and 6 mmol).

INFUSION SET

Refers to the hub, catheter, and insertion set.

INSERTION SET

The part of the infusion set inserted through the skin. It may be a fine metal needle or a larger metal needle, which is removed to leave a small teflon catheter under the skin.

INSULIN PUMP

A computerized, programmable device about the size of a beeper thatcan be programmed to send a continuous stream of insulin into the bloodstream as basal insulin, as well as larger amounts prior to meals as boluses. It replaces insulin injections. A pump delivers fast-acting insulin via a plastic catheter to either a teflon infusion set or a small metal needle inserted through the skin. Doses as small as 0.1 unit or less can be delivered with accuracy for gradual absorption into the bloodstream.

Insulin pumps cannot measure or control blood sugars on their own, but must be programmed based on information gained through frequent blood sugar monitoring.

RESERVOIR/SYRINGE/CARTRIDGE

A glass or plastic container which holds the fast-acting insulin inside the pump.

INTRODUCTION

If you're considering an insulin pump, beginning to use a pump, or already on a pump with less control than you desire, the answers to your questions are here. This book gives the information and in-depth detail you need for success on a pump. It can help any prospective pumper, any current pumper, and anyone who assists pumpers.

Pumping Insulin is for:

- Everyone considering or beginning to use an insulin pump
- Existing pumpers who want to improve their control
- Physicians, nurses, dieticians, physician assistants, nurse practitioners, and others who follow people on pumps
- Everyone who wants to end blood sugar highs and lows
- Everyone who wants to match insulin need with insulin delivery

Pumping Insulin tells you:

- What a pump is
- How to set up a pump
- How to chart and analyze your blood sugars
- How to count carbohydrates
- How to regulate basal rates and boluses for better control
- How to manage low blood sugars and high blood sugars
- How to minimize and solve pump problems
- How to feel better and live a healthier life
- When to seek help

This book provides step-by-step directions for setting and testing your pump, checklists for improving control, and specific examples of management techniques. Included are advanced blood sugar charting methods, carbohydrate counting instructions, approaches to exercise and pregnancy, specific directions for children and teens on pumps, and information on complications.

CHAPTER 1

Why Pumps Are Better

An insulin pump is the best tool available for achieving normal blood sugars. Pumping is preferred over injections by most health practitioners who have diabetes themselves because it most closely mimics the normal pancreas. Since the first published report of insulin pump use by Dr. Pickup in England in 1979,[1] the number of worldwide users has grown to around 100,000 people with Type 1 and Type 2 diabetes.

The rapid growth of pumps is due to the benefits that users experience and share with others. People on pumps have been the best advocates for pumping. Having a prominent individual like Nicole Johnson, Miss America for 1999, proudly wear an insulin pump raises the profile of pumpers and people with diabetes everywhere.

When an insulin pump is used well, a person feels better, lives more freely, and is likely to have fewer diabetes-related health problems as a result of improved blood sugar control. Pump wearers are happy because their insulin need is being met by insulin delivery in the right amount at the right time.

Those who use pumps say things like, "For the first time in years, I can eat when I want to," or "I can really control my blood sugars now, and I feel better, too." One enthusiastic supporter over the age of 70 who recently went on the pump told us, "The insecurity is gone. I feel so much more hopeful and positive about life. My control was good on injections according to my HbA1c, but I couldn't avoid overnight lows that created stress day after day. For the first time I really feel in control of things."

People with diabetes choose pumps for:

- a freer lifestyle
- improved HbA1c values
- better blood sugar control
- flexibility in meal timing and size

- fewer and less severe insulin reactions
- the ability to exercise without losing control
- control while travelling or working variable schedules
- membership in a community of forward-thinking, health-conscious people
- peace of mind

People on insulin pumps are often the most rewarding diabetes patients seen by health care providers. They are motivated problem-solvers wearing a tool that, when properly used, can keep their blood sugars in excellent control.

Health professionals recommend pumps for:

- managing the Dawn Phenomenon
- decreasing hypoglycemia
- reversing hypoglycemia unawareness
- preventing, delaying, or reversing complications
- improving control during the growth spurts of adolescence
- reducing wide blood sugar fluctuations in "brittle" diabetes
- delivering precise insulin doses for children and insulin-sensitive adults
- helping to stabilize erratic absorption of food in those with gastroparesis
- lessening insulin resistance in Type 2 diabetes
- tightening control during pregnancy

Pumps can help people who have peripheral or autonomic neuropathy,[2,3] early kidney disease (microalbuminuria),[4,5] and retinopathy.[6] Pumps are beneficial to those who have the Dawn Phenomenon, erratic control,[7,8] or insulin resistance.[9]

If you are deciding whether or not to use an insulin pump, consider the advantages it provides in controlling blood sugars, as well as its occasional drawbacks. **Pumping Insulin** covers these concerns and provides the tools needed to achieve excellent blood sugar control on a pump.

What's The Matter With Multiple Injections?

Many research studies, including the comprehensive Diabetes Control and Complications Trial (DCCT), have shown how important it is to keep blood sugars as normal as possible. For good control, a person with diabetes needs to match the amount of insulin required with the amount actually delivered by injection or a pump.

How is insulin delivered by a pump better than injected insulin? Injected insulin has three major problems. The action of long-acting insulins is unreliable, multiple injections are often inconvenient, and insulin from injections lacks specificity. This makes solving control problems more difficult.

Generally there are two lifestyle choices on injections that allow a person with diabetes to attempt to match insulin need with insulin delivery. One way is to live a very regulated life, control activities, give set doses of insulin, and eat the same amounts of carbohydrate at the same time every day. Variation in insulin absorption will continue, but most everything else is controlled. With this strictly regimented lifestyle, a person may have fairly good control with two injections or more. Before the days of flexible insulin therapy, it was assumed that a person with diabetes should, could, and would be willing to regiment his or her life to fixed doses of insulin and set meals and sacrifice freedom for good health. But experience has shown that most people simply will not or can not do this.

The other alternative is to live a varied lifestyle but adjust daily insulin doses accordingly. One diabetes specialist, Dr. Alan Marcus, states this clearly: "A basic tenet of diabetes care is that the degree of lifestyle flexibility that can be achieved is directly related to the number of daily insulin injections."[10] However, multiple injections of insulin will always be problematic in matching these normal daily insulin needs.

When you use injections, you use two insulins that work at different speeds. A fast insulin, like Humalog or Regular, is used to cover meals and is gone in three and a half to five hours. One of the long-acting insulins, such as Lente, NPH or Ultralente, is needed over long periods of time to keep the blood sugar from rising when you are not eating. To make this insulin available, a large pool of long-acting insulin is placed under the skin, to be absorbed gradually over the next 20 to 36 hours. Unfortunately, large pools of insulin like this can and frequently do create wide variations in the timing and amount of insulin actually absorbed into the blood.

Because two to three doses of long-acting insulin are needed each day and the timing of their onset of action and their strongest action varies from one day to the next, insulin peaks and valleys occur at different times each day. This variability throws off control, especially during exercise or when the skin is warmed by hot weather or a hot bath or sauna. In clinical studies, the amount of insulin that reaches a person's blood varies by 25% from one day to the next with injections.[11]

In an attempt to counter this problem, insulin companies are trying to produce long-acting insulins which have less peaking and a more consistent action from day to day. A new insulin called Lantus (glargine), designed to be a more consistent long-acting insulin, is now available. Lantus appears to lessen the unpredictability of long-acting insulins, and it shows a more constant, non-peaking 24-hour action. However, the variability between users continues and large day-to-day variations can occur with this insulin when the time at which the injection is taken varies, as it often does on weekends. Also, consistent-action insulins cannot match the variable background needs of someone with a Dawn Phenomenon or variable waking hours.

Peaking irregularity or a constant non-peaking action leads to another problem. Injections of long-acting insulin cannot be adjusted accurately enough to meet needs for more or less insulin at specific times. For example, insulin adjustments may be needed for the few hours causing the Dawn Phenomenon, or for a regularly scheduled hour of aerobic exercise.

Another problem with injections is inconvenience. Multiple daily injections often require at least four injections a day. Overcoming the inconvenience of this control program takes a great deal of motivation. A needle and insulin bottles or insulin pens have to be carried everywhere, to be taken out and used at restaurants or other public places. Although pens are relatively easy to carry and use, they have not gained wide acceptance in the United States and do not have the precision of a pump.

When you are on multiple injections and have control problems, you have a harder time sorting out which insulin is causing the problem. Long-acting and short-acting are mixed together in several injections a day. If your blood sugars are high or low, deciding whether the long-acting is peaking erratically or the short-acting given for a meal was the wrong amount becomes very confusing.

Contrast the difficulties of injections to using Humalog in a pump. Here, the insulin pool placed under the skin with each bolus is very small. Doses are calculated accurately in terms of background insulin and meal coverage. Daily variation in insulin delivery is reduced from 25% to about 3% because a pump avoids the unpredictable absorption problems that occur with the use of Lente, NPH, and Ultralente insulins.[12]

Obviously, the more precise and flexible an insulin delivery system, the better it meets needs and matches the demands of an active lifestyle. Pumps can deliver tenths of a unit of insulin at any time of day. They can be programmed to change the basal flow so that the blood sugar remains stable within the normal range overnight when a person is not eating, and also quickly adapt when a person increases his activity. A pump uses only short-acting, fast insulin, and the insulin delivery can be changed on a dime for spontaneous eating or exercise. Control problems are resolved by separately analyzing the effects of basals and boluses.

One of the major changes occurring today in diabetes is the shift toward continuous monitoring devices. These new monitors read blood sugars every 5 to 15 minutes which allows up or down trends in blood sugar readings to be quickly seen. Now more than ever, insulin need can be determined precisely. Devices like these make it even more important to have an insulin pump which can deliver small, precise doses and alter insulin delivery quickly to match need. When an insulin pump is used well, it is the best tool for achieving control while also allowing a freer lifestyle. Let's look more closely at factors that favor using a pump over injections.

Benefits Of Using A Pump

Match Your Insulin To Your Need

If you ask a person with Type 1 diabetes, "How much insulin do you take?" and she answers, "X units of this insulin and Y units of that insulin in the morning and X of this and Y of that in the evening," you can be sure she is not matching her insulin to her real need. But if she answers, "It depends," she is likely attempting to match insulin to need. This gives her a better chance of success in the game of blood sugar control.

"Is a pump any better than multiple injections for allowing a flexible lifestyle and promoting good control?" is the question most people ask when considering pump use. The discussion below details some of the differences between these two methods for optimizing flexibility and control.

In nondiabetic individuals, beta cells release precise amounts of insulin to cover two basic needs. First, the pancreas releases a background flow of insulin into the blood through the entire day. This background insulin directs the release and uptake by cells of glucose and fat as fuels. An insulin pump mimics this normal background release of insulin by means of its own background or basal insulin delivery.

Second, the normal pancreas releases short bursts or boluses of insulin into the bloodstream to match the carbohydrate content of food whenever it is eaten. This larger, quicker release is mimicked by meal boluses on a pump.

With diabetes, injected or pumped insulin must match three needs:

First, it must cover background insulin requirements. This "background or basal" insulin lets cells use the glucose made by the liver in the fasting state, controls the release of free fatty acids by liver and fat cells, balances other glucose-raising hormones found in the blood, transports certain amino acids into cells, and more.

Second, insulin must cover carbohydrates in foods.

Third, it must lower occasional high blood sugars to a normal range.

Meeting each of these needs requires precise insulin delivery. Most people on injections use two, three or more injections a day for accuracy. Using fewer injections is convenient, but it also means that insulin use is not defined clearly. When mixtures of short and long-acting insulins are used to cover all three needs, and the blood sugar is high or low, it becomes difficult to determine which need was poorly matched by which insulin. "My blood sugar's high. I don't know if I covered dinner with too little Humalog or if my NPH is too low," is a common dilemma.

In contrast, when a pump is used, small, precise boluses can be easily given at any time of day to cover food intake or occasional highs, while basal insulin is delivered automatically by the pump to cover the background needs determined earlier by the pump user.

When you use a pump, it becomes easier to recognize the source of an insulin dosing problem. Basal insulin delivery covers the background insulin requirements and keeps the blood sugar controlled when the user is not eating. The wearer can quickly test the basal rate on a pump by fasting overnight or by skipping a meal. When the blood sugar stays level or drops only slightly, the basal is correctly set.

The remainder of the insulin delivered by a pump is given as boluses. Boluses are infused over a short interval to meet the last two needs:

- covering carbohydrates, and
- lowering occasional high blood sugars.

On a pump, the basal insulin is always set and adjusted first until it keeps your blood sugars level while fasting. Once you've set and tested your basal rate, it's easy to determine if carb boluses are accurately balancing grams of carbohydrate you eat at a given time.

A correct ratio of insulin to carbs will keep post-meal blood sugars in a normal range with no lows or highs before the next meal. But if you incorrectly estimate a carb bolus using Humalog, a test of your blood sugar 2 hours after the meal will show an unwanted rise or fall. Because your basal rate has already been tested and you know it keeps your blood sugar level, you know immediately that your bolus for that particular meal needs to be adjusted. Of course, if your basal rate is not correctly set, you can't determine your boluses correctly.

If an occasional blood sugar is high, you can safely take a high blood sugar bolus that will bring it into your desired range based on the number of points (mg/dl) your blood sugar normally drops per unit of Humalog or Regular. Three and a half hours after giving a Humalog bolus to correct a high, the blood sugar would be normal if your basal is correctly set. This allows precise testing of the number of points your blood sugar drops per unit. Because insulin delivery from a pump is steadier and more predictable, you can more reliably correct high blood sugars.

Once carbohydrates are accurately covered and any high blood sugars corrected, the flow of basal insulin from the pump keeps the blood sugar within the desired range in the hours that follow. The precision of the pump in matching these three distinct needs makes good blood sugar control easier.

Live A Varied Lifestyle

Typical comments from new pumpers include: "I don't have to eat if I don't feel like it. I can wait till I'm hungry. It's the first time in years that I've felt hungry." or "It's given me freedom for the first time. I never thought it would make this much difference."

Few people live rigid, predictable lives. Work hours vary, meetings and events occur randomly, meals are delayed or missed, and eating is often done on the run. On weekends, people rise early or sleep late, and exercise more or less than usual and at different times of the day. Eating may include larger family or holiday meals or late dining after a movie.

Multiple Daily Injections (MDI), which involves testing the blood sugar at least four times a day and injecting at least four times, certainly allows a more flexible lifestyle than one or two injections, but a pump is the ideal tool for matching varied schedules. It's easy to eat a meal later than usual. With basal rates correctly set, a pumper can go all day without eating and maintain normal blood sugars. When carbs are eaten, a bolus can easily match that amount of carbohydrate.

If a blood sugar is high, insulin measured in fractions of a unit can be precisely delivered to lower the reading without having to prepare an extra injection. Before long periods of exercise, the basal rate can be reduced to prevent a low blood sugar. Extra carbohydrate may still be needed for the exercise, but fewer carbs are needed than if the insulin dose were not reduced. When you wear your pump, you are not tied to waking up or eating at set times of the day, nor will you find your blood sugars bouncing up and down as you meet the demands of an active life.

One large German study looked at how satisfied 77 people with Type 1 were when they switched from 1 or 2 injections a day to MDI, and at another group of 55 people who switched from MDI to an insulin pump. People on 1 or 2 injections who switched to MDI reported greater satisfaction with MDI. The level of satisfaction was even higher for the group who switched to insulin pump therapy. As insulin delivery becomes more sophisticated, users find that controlling their blood sugars has less impact on their lives. Pumps offer flexibility for leisure activities and create fewer problems with hypoglycemia. Even weekend or vacation blood sugars are significantly improved with a pump.[13]

Correct High Morning Blood Sugars

The first blood sugar of the day is usually the most important one for controlling the entire day's readings. "If I wake up high, my whole day is shot!" is a typical complaint because an early morning high is often quite difficult to bring down through the day.

Some 50% to 70% of people with Type 1 diabetes find they need more insulin in the early morning hours to offset a rise in blood sugar.[14] This rise, called the Dawn Phenomenon, is created by a normal increase in the production and release of growth hormone, and to a lesser extent by cortisol and adrenaline, which trigger the production and release of glucose from the liver. If this need is not met by an increase in insulin delivery, the blood sugar rises as daylight approaches and is high when the person awakens.

A typical adjustment for a person with a Dawn Phenomenon usually provides slightly less basal insulin during the middle of the night when insulin sensitivity is highest, and slightly more basal insulin before and during the Dawn Phenomenon.

An equal or even larger percentage of people with Type 2 diabetes find their pre-breakfast reading is the hardest of the day to control. Even though their problem also occurs at dawn, the source of the problem is different from the Dawn Phenomenon. Most people with Type 2 have an excess of fat cells in the abdomen, referred to as an apple shape. During the night, these fat cells release fat, which is picked up by the portal vein going to the liver. This fat makes the liver less sensitive to the insulin passing by.

Because of this insulin resistance, more insulin is needed to do the job of stopping the liver in its production and release of glucose. If insulin production fails to keep up with the rising need because of ageing and weight gain, the liver will make more and more unneeded glucose during the night. For people with Type 2, an insulin pump is the ideal way to deliver the precise, small insulin doses needed to stop the liver from increasing glucose production.

People who have a strong Dawn Phenomenon or an unruly liver find that it's difficult to control the morning blood sugar with any injected insulin regimen. On a pump, however, controlling the morning blood sugar becomes a simple insulin adjustment. The basal rate can be adjusted precisely to prevent the blood sugar from rising during the night. Easy programming allows each pumper to set basal rates to meet individual needs at each hour. "I usually wake up in the morning with a normal blood sugar!" is a joy shared by many new pumpers.

Prevent Frequent And Severe Insulin Reactions

Insulin reactions are the most frightening part of diabetes control. People may avoid tight control to avoid insulin reactions; they also may not check their blood sugars in order to avoid seeing how high they are running. Failing to check blood sugars makes control impossible. Another common problem comes from taking too much insulin to bring highs down, which leads to subsequent low blood sugars and erratic control.

Fewer insulin reactions occur with an insulin pump when it is set up correctly because it delivers insulin more precisely and conveniently. It better matches doses to needs: basal for background need, and boluses for carbohydrates and high blood sugars. It delivers basal insulin as tiny droplets of a fast-absorbing insulin for quicker insulin

> ### Pumps Excel At Control
>
> Because a pump gives precise insulin delivery, most people can achieve normal blood sugars most of the time. On a pump, always realize that if your blood sugars frequently run high or low, your current basal rates or boluses need to be adjusted to better fit your lifestyle.

response. The precision of both basal and bolus insulin delivery is especially helpful for people who are sensitive to insulin or who need less than 30 to 35 units a day. Erratic peaks of injected long-acting insulin that cause lows are avoided entirely.

Another benefit noted by many who use pumps is that when an insulin reaction does occur, it is usually less severe. Because insulin delivery better matches need, the blood sugar drops more slowly, giving the pump wearer extra time to recognize the symptoms of a low blood sugar. As reaction time lengthens, it becomes easier to remedy a reaction before it becomes severe.

Prevent And Control Complications

Fear of complications related to diabetes is another reason to consider an insulin pump. All of the complications associated with diabetes---neuropathy, nephropathy, retinopathy, and to some extent heart problems---develop in the presence of high blood sugars. Control your blood sugar better and you reduce your risk for complications. Of course, controlling other risk factors is also important for slowing or reversing complications. Reducing fat and protein intake, lowering elevated blood pressure, exercising, improving diet, avoiding smoking, and controlling cholesterol levels have all shown benefits. Maintaining normal blood sugar levels is the ideal way to prevent complications, however.

Blood sugar control becomes easier, more systematic, and more understandable when using a pump. Having a better handle on blood sugar control increases motivation and inspires those on pumps to use them for a healthier life. If complications are present when pump therapy is started, they can often be stabilized or reversed. Further damage is frequently avoided because of the improved control on a pump.

What's A "Normal" Reading?

Normal readings will be slightly different depending on where the glucose is drawn from to be measured. Most blood sugar meters measure glucose either in whole blood or in plasma. Plasma readings, like the lab values at your doctor's office, are about 10% higher than whole blood readings.

Many new meters and most of the continuous blood sugar monitors measure glucose in interstitial fluid. These readings are about 10% lower than whole blood. Some meters are also switch-hitters that apply an adjustment factor to translate the reading into a whole blood value. Be sure you know what your glucose is measured in, as this can change how you interpret your readings.

	Typical normal values before and after eating when measuring glucose in:		
	Interstitial Fluid	**Whole Blood**	**Plasma**
Before Meals	90 mg/dl or less (5 mmol)	100 mg/dl or less (5.6 mmol)	110 mg/dl or less (6.1 mmol)
2 hrs After Meals	120 mg/dl or less (6.7 mmol)	130 mg/dl or less (7.2 mmol)	140 mg/dl or less (7.8 mmol)

What About Type 2 Diabetes?

While insulin pumps have been used primarily by people with Type 1 diabetes, the number of people with Type 2 diabetes who use pumps is growing. With Type 1 diabetes, an outside source of insulin is needed for life, and the benefit of an insulin pump is rather obvious.

In contrast, Type 2 diabetes is usually caused by insulin resistance, with insulin production often continuing at normal or even elevated levels for several years. Extra insulin is needed to overcome resistance to insulin. The stress of overproduction, along with the toxic effects of excess glucose and free fatty acids, may cause beta cells to gradually stop producing insulin.

As already noted, a major control problem often seen with Type 2 is the high blood sugar encountered on waking in the morning, even after going to bed with a normal reading. The blood sugar rises during the night as the liver makes and releases glucose into the bloodstream when it does not "sense" insulin, because it is resistant to insulin. Higher blood sugars create even more insulin resistance, and the beta cells cannot keep up.

An insulin pump is ideal for delivering the extra nighttime insulin at exactly the time when it is needed. Often insulin doses and circulating insulin levels are cut in half because of the precision of the pump. A pump is also ideal for bolusing for meals and snacks. Matching insulin need to delivery means that the blood sugars are better controlled at the same time less insulin is needed. Weight loss often needed with Type 2 diabetes is easier because the person is not eating to avoid lows and can easily reduce calorie intake by simply taking smaller boluses.

Though rarely the first treatment option considered, insulin pumps have the following distinct advantages for those with Type 2 diabetes who use insulin:

- Blood sugar control is improved with less insulin due to the more natural delivery of insulin. The resulting lower blood insulin levels and improved control create greater sensitivity to insulin so that even less insulin becomes needed for control.

- Similar to the DCCT findings in Type 1 studies, diabetes complications are greatly reduced in Type 2 diabetes as blood sugar control is improved.[15]

- Weight loss is easier because calorie intake can be balanced with bolus reductions, eliminating the need to overeat to compensate for excess insulin.

- Triglyceride levels, which cause high cholesterol and excess clotting, are often dangerously high in Type 2 diabetes, but a pump can lower them through its efficient use of a fast insulin in boluses calculated to cover each meal.[15,16]

- Fasting blood sugars are much easier to control.[15,16]

Some older people diagnosed as Type 2 are actually slow onset Type 1s. Although older than most Type 1s, they are slender and sensitive to insulin. They often produce their own insulin for several years and can benefit from using a device that will deliver the small doses of insulin they require.

It should be stressed that normal blood sugars benefit all types of diabetes. Whether a person has Type 1 or 2, high blood sugars cause damage. If weight loss or an increase in activity occurs, basal rates and boluses may need to be reduced rapidly. Extra testing is vital whenever these lifestyle changes are underway.

Research studies also suggest that even a few days' treatment with an insulin pump can be of great benefit in Type 2 diabetes. In one French study, 82 people who were unable to control their blood sugars with a low calorie diet and maximum doses of Glucophage (metformin) were temporarily placed on insulin pumps for periods of 8 to 32 days. Blood sugars rapidly improved at the start of pump therapy, but even more interesting, their control continued to be improved after the pump treatment stopped! This brief "vacation" appears to allow an overworked pancreas to once again produce the insulin required for several months after this brief period of pump use.[17]

A Turkish study tried the same approach--2 weeks of pump treatment--for people with newly-diagnosed Type 2 diabetes who did not respond to diet control. As a result of temporary insulin pump use, six of the original 13 patients were able to stay well controlled on diet alone for 16 to 59 months at the time of the report, although four people required a second two-week treatment, and one required a third treatment.[18]

Are There Drawbacks?

Ketoacidosis

Although long-acting insulins can create insulin absorption problems, they have one advantage--their long period of action can protect against ketoacidosis, which occurs in people who produce little or no insulin. Injecting long-acting insulin creates a pool under the skin that will release insulin over the next 24 hours for NPH or Lente insulins or over the next 30 hours for Ultralente. On a pump, a much smaller pool of Humalog or Regular insulin is deposited under the skin. If insulin delivery from a pump is interrupted for any reason, this small pool of fast insulin is quickly used and blood sugars can start to rise 90 minutes later. In about three hours the level of insulin in the blood may drop to 60% of what it was originally.

When the insulin level drops, cells can't get glucose for fuel and must convert to using fat. As more and more fat is consumed, by-products called ketones begin to rise in the blood. After approximately four hours with no delivery of Humalog, a danger-ous acidic state called ketoacidosis occurs.[19] In studies done in the early 1980s, ketoaci-dosis requiring an emergency room or hospital visit occurred once in every six and a half years of pump use.[20] Since these early studies, advances in pump therapy have decreased the risk for ketoacidosis.[21] Even so, ketoacidosis remains more likely on a pump than with injections. In seven more recent research studies that looked at the risk of ketoacidosis on pumps between 1985 and 1990, ketoacidosis occurs once for every 10 to 25 years of pump use.[22]

Insulin Reactions

The Diabetes Control and Complications Trial (DCCT) ending in 1993 clearly showed that an increased risk for insulin reactions was the major drawback when tightening blood sugar control. This increased risk occurred when either multiple

What About My Eyes?

If you have moderate background retinopathy or a more severe case, this eye damage may temporarily worsen when you start on a pump. This tendency for existing eye damage to worsen is believed to be triggered by a temporary rise in vascular endothelial growth factor (VEGF) levels, in association with high levels of protein kinase C (PKC). These factors cause the growth of new blood vessels. Angiogenesis inhibitors, so-called because they reduce the formation of new blood vessels, are now being tested in clinical trials. These drugs may be able to prevent and treat diabetic retinopathy.

If you have any existing retinopathy, you should be followed by an experienced ophthalmologist to prevent eye damage or treat any that may worsen during early pump use.[23,24] After 6 to 12 months of good control, retinopathy often stabilizes and may slowly improve, but see your ophthalmologist to verify this.

If your blood sugar control has not been great, your physician may also advise that you gradually improve your control during the first few weeks on the pump so that less VEGF is released. Another approach is to use high doses of vitamin E for the first few months. Usually 1,200 or 1,500 units a day is needed to reduce PKC which corrects abnormal blood flow.[25, 26, 27, 28] The reduction in PKC appears to block much of the damage caused by VEGF.

injections or an insulin pump was being used to improve control. Severe insulin reactions, requiring the assistance of another person, occurred three times more often in the intensive control group than in the traditional control group.

Severe hypoglycemia occurred 62 times in 100 patient-years, or once every 18 months on average in the intensive group compared to 19 times in 100 patient years in the control group.[29] Episodes of coma or seizure occurred 16 times per 100 patient-years in the intensive group compared to 5 times in the control group. Some participants had multiple episodes, while many others had none at all.

In a more recent study conducted in 1998, Disetronic surveyed an international group of 6,890 pump users from the US, Germany, the Netherlands, and Austria. Respondents had diabetes an average of 21 years. Fifty percent had been on the pump 0-2 years, another 30% for 3-5 years, 15% for 6-10 years, and the rest up to 15 years. When this large group of pump users compared pumps to their previous injections, 62% reported that their hypoglycemia was less frequent, 17% reported it as more frequent, and 21% said it was about the same.

The overall benefits of improved blood sugar control with more precise insulin dosing are believed to greatly outweigh the disadvantages caused by an increased risk of hypoglycemia for most people with diabetes. Careful, consistent monitoring will significantly lower the risk of lows, especially when blood sugar patterns are recognized and acted upon before symptoms become severe. The new continuous monitors, with warning alarms set at desired thresholds, may eliminate the risk of lows as they become more available.

Hypoglycemia Unawareness

Low blood sugars with little or no warning occur in some people who have diabetes. When a person requires the assistance of someone else to recognize and correct a low blood sugar, he/she has a condition called hypoglycemia unawareness. It is more likely to occur in those who have had diabetes for a number of years, especially after having several low blood sugars over a short period of time. Lows can be triggered by skipping a meal after having taken a bolus for it, after excess alcohol, or after increased or unusual activity. However, most situations in which frequent lows are occurring are caused by giving too much insulin. Hypoglycemia unawareness can be a danger to those who have it and a problem for those around the person, especially if he or she is convinced there is no problem and refuses treatment.

Hypoglycemia unawareness may occur more easily when using an insulin pump because fewer warning symptoms occur when the blood sugar drops gradually. When a person starts on a pump, the risk for insulin reactions is about the same as when attempting tight control with injections, but as experience grows, reactions usually become both less frequent and less severe.[30] Most episodes of hypoglycemia unawareness occur during sleep, and pumps are excellent at delivering the precise nighttime basal rates that can help to prevent these lows.

Because a pump gradually lessens the risk of hypoglycemia, it will also lessen the occurrence of hypoglycemia unawareness.[31] In one large study of 225 pumpers in Atlanta, the frequency of hypoglycemia was compared in the first year of pump use to the previous year on MDI. Severe hypoglycemia dropped from 138 events for every 100 years of use with MDI to 22 events in the first year on pumps. The lower rates continued with 26 events in the second year of pump use, 39 in the third, and 36 in the fourth.[30] As blood sugars become better controlled on a pump, the risk of reactions is lessened, and should one occur, a pumper has more time to recognize the symptoms and correct the blood sugar, even though symptoms may be milder. The combination of these factors in most cases will reduce the risk of hypoglycemia unawareness.

Pumping may, in fact, reverse hypoglycemia unawareness. Irl Hirsch, M.D. and Ruth Farkas-Hirsch, R.N., who follow a large group of people on insulin pumps in Seattle, say, "since insulin absorption is more predictable, hypoglycemia unawareness should be considered an important indication for an insulin pump."[32] The improved cell metabolism that results from carefully patterned insulin delivery on a pump allows cells to repair and cell function to improve. A reduction in the frequency of low blood sugars allows a person to regain awareness of his/her own reactions.[33] It is estimated that one in five people with Type 1 diabetes currently has hypoglycemia unawareness. More information is provided in Chapter 16 on how to reverse it.

If you have ever become unconscious or incoherent due to a low blood sugar and required the assistance of someone else to treat this reaction, discuss this carefully with your physician. Your insulin pump therapist can help you manage and avoid this dangerous situation.

Site Infections And Abscesses

Skin is a natural defense against infection. When an infusion set is placed through the skin, it breaks this protection and offers an open door to bacteria. Skin infections are almost never seen with injections, but the risk for infections increases on a pump.

If an infection occurs, an antibiotic may be needed. If the infection progresses to an abscess, the abscess must be lanced and drained. If the infection is severe or does not respond to treatment, hospitalization may be required. The use of good hygiene, covered in Chapter 5, can reduce the risk of infection to a great extent.

Self Image

Many people experience doubts about wearing a pump before they put it on. Attachment to a pump may seem inconvenient, annoying, and potentially embarrassing. Even though today's beeper-sized pumps weigh only a few ounces and are very portable, physical attachment to a small computerized device may seem intolerable.

Although a pump always goes with you on a belt, in a pocket or under your clothes, detachment is relatively easy with today's infusion sets. However, time off the pump is usually limited to one hour with no pre-detachment bolus, or three hours when a bolus is given before detaching to replace the basal insulin that will be missed.

Some people have difficulty accepting this type of attachment, especially if they feel other people will see this and consider them as different or as having a "disease." The teen years and early twenties are particularly difficult ages to be different, and the perceived stigma of a pump may make its use impractical at these ages.

Another reason for deciding not to use a pump is active involvement in contact sports. Here the presence of an external, but attached device can sometimes present problems. Sports problems can often be worked out through easy detachment of infusion sets.

After attaching a pump, however, people are almost always surprised at its comfort and wearability. The feared personal rejection becomes instead the respect of friends and relatives as they realize you are taking advantage of advanced technology to control your blood sugar better.

If you have concerns about these issues, and many people do, see whether you can obtain a nonoperating loaner pump to try out from your physician/health care team. Remember: for very little inconvenience, using a pump will probably improve and prolong the quality of your life. A comment heard frequently from new pumpers is that, "My friends (family, co-workers) say that I look healthier and more alert."

Summary

Pumps provide distinct advantages in the control of blood sugars. When they are set up appropriately and used well, they allow more consistent, responsive and precise delivery of insulin so that blood sugars closer to normal are maintained. As blood sugars improve, the chance of developing health problems related to diabetes lessens. Some research studies have shown that good control, which may be best gained by pump use, can even reverse diabetes-related complications.

An informed person on a correctly-set pump approximates normal daily life without diabetes. Pumpers can skip meals, eat late, and cover variations in carbohydrate intake. Quick adjustments can be made whenever elevated blood sugars, exercise, or unexpected illnesses occur.

Because a pump closely copies the function of the pancreas, it creates freedom for the person wearing it. This may sound like a frivolous reason to someone who does not have diabetes, but to someone who has had to eat meals on a rigid schedule, who must have a carbohydrate snack every night before bed, who occasionally wakes up in a soaking sweat at 3 a.m., who faces high blood sugars every morning, who suffers from lows when exercising, who feels restrained from eating spontaneously, who has returned to consciousness in an emergency room with an intravenous catheter in one arm, or who simply wants to sleep late on the weekend, wearing a pump can mean a pleasurable life again! Having diabetes should not end the ability to live a normal life.

Pumps do have some drawbacks. The risk of ketoacidosis is increased, as is the incidence of skin infections. Constant attachment to an external device can be a perceived drawback or a real one if the wearer participates in certain sports such as football or soccer, or is in an occupation such as lifeguard or belly dancer. The drawbacks are manageable with constant attention and good technique.

A pump has more advantages than drawbacks, but a pump is only a tool. As a tool, it is only as successful as the abilities and efforts of the person responsible for its use. The basic requirements for success demanded of the pump user and health professional are given in the text box on the next page. The information in this book is designed to enable your success on a pump.

When all the advantages and drawbacks are carefully weighed, a pump clearly offers most people an advantage in their quest for a healthy lifestyle with normal blood sugars.

Health Care Provider/Pumper Requirements For Success On A Pump

Health care provider will

- train the pumper in good technical skills for pump use
- teach problem-solving skills so that the pump user can take charge of day-to-day blood sugar control
- set starting basals and boluses and help to test and adjust them
- gradually train a capable pump user in complete blood sugar management with a pump

Pumper will

- count carbs or use an equivalent diet method, and record food eaten
- test and record blood sugar readings and insulin reactions
- test basals and boluses
- learn to match basals and boluses to their insulin need by problem-solving blood sugar patterns
- learn and use good technique in handling technical aspects of pumping

"An optimist is a fellow who believes a housefly is looking for a way out."

George Jean Nathan

PumpFormance Checklist

A primary concern for all pumpers is, "How do I get the most out of my pump? Since I'm investing time and money in this technology, how can I be sure I'm getting the best control?" Although the pump offers today's most advanced approach to blood sugar control, a pump user has to know how to set up, test, and modify insulin delivery. For complete success, basal rates and boluses need to be adjusted to adapt to changes in daily life. The ability to problem-solve when blood sugar problems arise is critical.

The PumpFormance Checklist below sets goals for optimum pump use. If you're beginning to use a pump, look at the Checklist to see the level of control you are working toward. If you are already on a pump, review each question to assess your level of control and where it can be improved. If you're a physician or health care provider, use these questions to help set realistic goals with the pump users you assist.

How well is your pump tuned? Answer the questions below in the order given. If you answer "yes", go to the next question. If "no", look to the right for the **Pumping Insulin** chapter that applies, and correct your control with your doctor's help before proceeding. For example, if your basal rates are incorrectly set, it won't be possible to set boluses correctly until this is remedied. Each "No" directs you to sections in the book for steps to correct this problem.

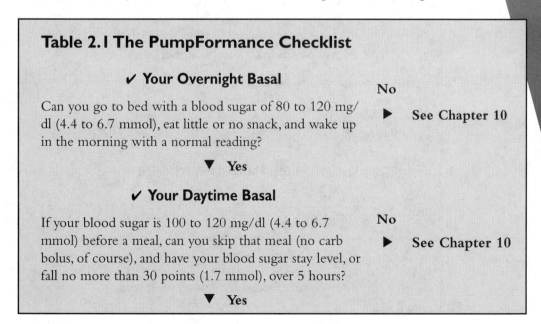

Table 2.1 The PumpFormance Checklist

✔ **Your Overnight Basal**

Can you go to bed with a blood sugar of 80 to 120 mg/dl (4.4 to 6.7 mmol), eat little or no snack, and wake up in the morning with a normal reading?

No ▶ **See Chapter 10**

▼ Yes

✔ **Your Daytime Basal**

If your blood sugar is 100 to 120 mg/dl (4.4 to 6.7 mmol) before a meal, can you skip that meal (no carb bolus, of course), and have your blood sugar stay level, or fall no more than 30 points (1.7 mmol), over 5 hours?

No ▶ **See Chapter 10**

▼ Yes

✔ Your Use Of Carb Counting

Can you determine the grams of carbohydrate in foods you are eating, either through carb counting, food exchanges, or by using another dietary system?

No
▶ See Chapter 7

▼ Yes

✔ Your Use Of Carb Boluses

With a normal blood sugar before a meal, can you cover the carbohydrate in the meal with a carb bolus so that your blood sugar is normal 4 hours later?

No
▶ See Chapter 11

▼ Yes

✔ Your Use Of High Blood Sugar Boluses

When you have a high blood sugar, can you take a high blood sugar bolus to bring your blood sugar to normal 4 hours later?

No
▶ See Chapter 12

▼ Yes

✔ Your Determination Of Unused Boluses

When you give 2 or more boluses within 3.5 hours of each other, do you know how to determine how much insulin has yet to work in order to avoid reactions, or if an additional bolus is needed?

No
▶ See Chapter 13

▼ Yes

✔ How You Handle Insulin Reactions

When you have a low blood sugar, can you recognize and handle it by yourself, and keep your blood sugar from bouncing above 150 mg/dl (8.3 mmol) afterward?

No
▶ See Chapter 15

▼ Yes

✔ How You Handle Exercise

When you exercise, can you avoid severe reactions and keep your blood sugar between 70 and 150 mg/dl (3.9 to 8.3 mmol)?

No
▶ See Chapter 19

▼ Yes

Terrific! No problems! Check again later!

Why Normal Blood Sugars?

Keeping your blood sugars relatively normal is the greatest and most important challenge you face with diabetes. This book provides you with the information, tools, and motivation needed to take on this challenge and succeed. This chapter reviews the importance of near-normal, stable blood sugars. Future chapters provide practical ways to successfully meet the challenge.

In this chapter, we'll discuss

- The benefits of controlling your blood sugar
- How high blood sugars can cause complications
- Ways to prevent and deal with complications

Is Testing Enough?

You may often think, "I test my blood sugars. I'm doing enough." But let's see what the DCCT found. At the start of the DCCT in the mid-1980s, the conventional group used urine testing and one or two injections a day. But by the end of the study in 1993, 83 percent of this conventional group were testing blood sugars several times a day and 91 percent were on two injections a day.[23] Unfortunately, even though they had improved their therapy, their blood sugar control did not improve! Merely testing more often had no effect on their control, although without self-testing, no improvement would be possible.

A major lesson from this landmark study, and from other similar research findings, is that testing blood sugars is not enough. You must use your readings to adjust the things that really affect your blood sugar, such as insulin doses and carbohydrate intake. You are likely to need expert coaching and advice before you see any improvement in your blood sugar. Testing lays a foundation for controlling your blood sugars, but regular visits to your diabetes clinic and your own involvement in your care speeds up your progress to better control.

What Causes Complications?

Why do high blood sugars cause complications? Damage always begins at the molecular level, and then spreads to larger structures like cells. When a large number of cells have been damaged, damage appears in organs like the eyes, kidneys and nerves.

What causes damage to start? Cell health depends on a steady supply of fuel from glucose and free fatty acids. These fuels are regulated by insulin released directly into the blood from beta cells in the pancreas. When insulin levels are low, glucose builds up in the blood because it has a difficult time entering the cells of certain organs. Furthermore, the liver releases excess glucose into the bloodstream. If any food is eaten, the blood sugar rises even higher.

High blood sugars indicate that cells dependant on insulin are not receiving fuel properly. Other types of cells have high internal glucose levels and cannot perform their normal functions. Routine repair processes cannot be performed as well. Key enzymes become damaged and manufacture fewer of their essential products. This strain and functional breakdown over a period of time results in widespread organ damage.

Low blood sugars are also destructive. When blood sugars are low, certain cells, particularly brain and nerve cells, encounter trouble because they depend exclusively on glucose for fuel, and now they can't get it. Many clinicians believe that erratic control, with blood sugars swinging from high to low and back, adds to the physical damage found in diabetes complications.

The impact of a high blood sugar environment on the development of complications is illustrated by studies of transplanted kidneys. When a kidney is taken from someone without diabetes and transplanted into someone with diabetes, the blood sugars must be controlled or kidney damage typical of diabetes will develop in this nondiabetic kidney. Damage is caused by the high blood sugar environment into which it is placed, not by the composition of the kidney itself. Some patients are lucky enough to receive a combined kidney and pancreas transplant at the same time. If they maintain normal blood sugars, they will have no damage to their kidneys for periods as long as 10 years in this diabetes-free environment.

Of particular interest is the fact that high blood sugars cause damage only to certain cells. What makes some cells prone to damage while little damage occurs in others? The cells in the eyes, kidneys, heart, blood vessels, and nervous system are most prone to damage because they pick up glucose directly from the blood without using insulin. This automatically exposes them to high internal levels of glucose whenever the blood sugar is high. Other cells require insulin to pick up glucose, and these cells are not as prone to damage.

Do high blood sugars always lead to complications? Not necessarily. Some people escape serious health problems despite poor blood sugar control, but many people with poor blood sugar control will develop one or more of the complications typical of diabetes, involving the eyes, kidneys, nerves, and blood vessels. Often, factors like genetics, nutrition, exercise, blood pressure, smoking, alcohol intake, hormone levels, vitamin and mineral balance, and stress levels determine the extent of damage. The most important thing to remember is that diabetes complications do not occur in people without diabetes because their blood sugars remain normal. The world contains an excellent control group with several billion individuals who never develop any diabetes complications because their blood sugars are normal.

Can You Prevent Complications?

One benefit of keeping sugars normal, clearly demonstrated in thousands of research studies, is that the risk for developing serious complications like kidney failure, blindness, and nerve damage is greatly reduced. Furthermore, research suggests that normal blood sugars also protect against cardiovascular problems, such as heart attacks and strokes. People with poorly controlled blood sugars are at higher risk for heart disease, partly because high blood sugars lead to higher cholesterol levels, especially higher triglycerides.

One of the most important studies of diabetes in recent years, the DCCT, provided invaluable information on the benefits of normal blood sugars. This extensive nine-year study that cost $167 million was completed in 1993.

In the study, a group of 1,441 people with Type 1 diabetes were followed for three to nine years. Half were randomly assigned to a "control" group in which blood sugars were conventionally controlled on one or two injections a day. The other half were assigned to an intensive control group, with the task of keeping their blood sugars as normal as possible using three or more injections a day or an insulin pump.

Table 3.1 HbA1c Shows Risk For Severe Eye Damage[34]	
HbA1c lab nl = 5.4%-7.4%	**Risk of Severe Eye Damage**
6.2-8.3%	1.0
8.4-9.0%	5.3 X higher
9.1-9.8%	16.4 X higher
9.9-13.6%	26.1 X higher

The DCCT validated that better blood sugars lead to improved health. Many researchers had long suspected this, but the remarkable finding was how much the risk of complications was reduced. Compared to the conventional control group, the intensive control group experienced up to 76 percent less eye damage, 54 percent less kidney disease and 60 percent less nerve damage.[29] This protective effect occurred even though the intensive control group did not keep their blood sugars totally within a normal range.

Conclusions similar to the DCCT results for Type 1 diabetes were drawn in a large study of people with Type 2 diabetes at Kumamoto University Medical School in Japan.[35] It has become clear that high blood sugars cause damage no matter what type of diabetes you have.

Table 3.2 BG Control In Last Year Affects Eyes	
HbA1c in the previous year (nl = 4.2% to 5.6%)	Percentage whose eye disease worsened
less than 6.13%	9.5%
6.13-7.35%	18.6%
over 7.35%	33%
Adapted from Chantelau et. al.[37]	

Since damage to the eyes, nerves, and kidneys is similar in both types of diabetes, the underlying cause is presumed to be the same.

The DCCT also showed that there is a direct relationship between how high your blood sugars are and your risk of complications. The higher your HbA1c, the greater your risk for complications. In addition, there is a strong suspicion among clinical researchers that the degree to which the blood sugars vary and how long they are high also are factors in determining cell and organ damage.

The DCCT and Kumamoto studies demonstrate that optimal glycemic control with intensive insulin therapy prevents the onset and delays the progression of eye, kidney, and nerve damage. The glycemic thresholds which seem to prevent complications from starting or progressing in the Kumamoto study were a HbA1c value below 6.5%, fasting blood sugars below 110 mg/dl, and 2 hours after a meal blood sugars below 180 mg/dl. Most diabetes specialists try to keep the HbA1c no higher than 1% above the lab's upper limit for normal. In other words, if the normal range for the HbA1c at your lab is 4 to 6%, your HbA1c should be no higher than 7%.

Can Complications Be Reversed?

Keeping your blood sugars normal prevents complications, but what if you already have one or more complications? Complications that are at a low to moderate degree of damage appear to be reversible.

For instance, one study in Oslo, Norway, of people with existing complications compared a control group using conventional therapy of two shots a day with another group using an insulin pump or five or six injections a day. On tests of nerve function, the intensive group, and pump users in particular, showed no further deterioration of nerve function at one year. At two years, they showed a slight improvement, and this improvement continued over three years and four years of improved control.[5] Kidney function also improved, but only after four years.[36] Today, there are a wide variety of medications, growth factors, nutrients, and physical interventions that are being tested to prevent and repair organ damage.

There are obvious limits to reversing damage. Some cells, like those in the eye and kidney, can't be regenerated or repaired once damage becomes severe. If a cell in the eye has been destroyed, vision cannot be restored to that area. If an eye cell is only partially damaged, however, indications are that the body may be able to restore some of the lost function.

How long does it take for good control to reverse damage? In contrast to the Norway study, most studies of interventions for kidney disease often show immediate results, while repairing nerve damage takes longer. New nerve growth factors, now in clinical trials, may soon speed nerve repair.

The outlook for improvement as blood sugar control is normalized may be similar to that for a person who stops smoking. Once a smoker stops, it takes about seven years for the ex-smoker's health risks to equal those of a nonsmoker. A similar time-table for overcoming physical damage from uncontrolled diabetes is likely.

Any improvement you make in your blood sugar control lessens damage. If blood sugars are normalized, some damage appears to be reversible. The extent to which existing damage can be reversed is in early stages of testing at this time.

Summary

Blood sugar control is the most important way to prevent or repair organ damage. Other factors are involved, but none is as important as blood sugar control. So the answer to "Why should I keep blood sugars normal?" is "To stay healthy and avoid complications."

Is improved health enough motivation to take on the challenge of blood sugar control? We hope so. Not only will tomorrow's health outcome look rosier, but you start feeling better immediately as you begin to master your blood sugars on an insulin pump. The improved sense of well-being and quality of life that can come from stable and normal blood sugars is an important motivation for many to start pumping.[38]

The chapters that follow provide the motivated reader with the tools to use the pump well in order to improve their control, reduce blood sugar swings, feel better, and prevent or reverse complications.

Liberty means responsibility. That is why most men dread it.

George Bernard Shaw

Are You A Candidate For A Pump?

CHAPTER 4

Successful pumping takes commitment, skills, and knowledge. Consider the important questions below before making your decision about an insulin pump. You may also want to review this list if problems continue to arise while on a pump. Although the questions are focused on the person who will be wearing the pump, they should also be considered by the health care personnel, spouses, parents, and other support people who will be involved in the day-to-day results of pump use.

Consider

- Why are you interested in starting on a pump?

- What are your goals for pump therapy?

- Who initially brought up the idea of pumping?

- Do you believe that you can control your blood sugars, and that your day-to-day control of blood sugars affects your health?

- Are your current and long-term pump goals realistic?

- How will an insulin pump fit into your daily life?

- Are there special situations you need to consider: athletics, work environment, social events, etc.?

- Have you accepted your diabetes? For example, do you remember to wear your medical ID tag? Are you comfortable testing your blood sugar in front of other people?

The authors want to give special thanks to Barb Schreiner, R.N. M.N., C.D.E. and Shannon Brow, R.N., B.S., C.D.E. for their contributions to this chapter and the next one.

- Are you self-conscious about your body? Will wearing a pump be an uncomfortable sign of having diabetes? Will others accept you as readily if you are on a pump?

- What other blood sugar control programs have you tried? Insulin pen? Multiple daily injections?

- Who have you talked with about the pump? Do you know anyone using one?

- How do you measure the impact food has on your blood sugars---carb counting, exchanges, or some other method?

- How often do you monitor your blood sugar? Are you consistent about testing and recording your results?

- Do you make adjustments in your insulin doses or food based on your test results?

- How effective is your current control? What is your most recent HbA1c?

- What has been your experience with hypoglycemia? Any severe hypoglycemia? Any hypoglycemia unawareness?

- Who will you call if problems arise?

- Do you have confidence that pumps are safe?

- If you have arthritis in your hands, can you punch the pump buttons, fill the reservoir, and place the infusion set?

- What will be your out-of-pocket costs for pump therapy? Do these fit into your budget? What if your insurance company or HMO refuses to cover the cost?

Questions for parents of a child or teen who is considering the pump:

- Why does your child or teen want to try pump therapy? How do you know?

- How much involvement should you as the parent have in this program? How do you feel about your child or teen taking care of his/her diabetes?

- Will you have access to a trained diabetes professional when you need help?

Your answers to these questions should be considered carefully before deciding to start on a pump. Not everyone is a good pump candidate. You should say "no" if this therapy does not fit your desires or lifestyle.

Things To Consider

If you are convinced pumping is for you, the next step is to select a pump and try different infusion sets. Each type of pump available in the United States has features that appeal to different needs and individuals.

Prior to selecting a pump, it is important to watch the manufacturer's videotape, handle the device, push the buttons, and generally become familiar with the pump's features. This can be done by contacting your diabetes educator or sales representatives for the pump manufacturers.

When selecting an insulin pump, consider the following:

- How low can the basal rate be programmed, how frequently does basal delivery occur, and is the pump motor strong enough to avoid clogging at low basal rates? This is important for children and thin or insulin-sensitive adults, who often require low basal rates.

- How easy is it to program and use this pump?

- How are batteries changed? Where will you get replacement batteries and how often are they needed?

- How easy is it to stop a bolus? If the pump is for a child, can a caregiver easily learn to stop the pump in an emergency?

- How much information is stored in the pump's memory? This is an important feature if the user may be distracted at mealtimes, if there is a concern about the overlapping of boluses, or if parents want to verify pump use by their child or teen.

- Can the pump be used or detached easily during sports and other activities?

- If you participate in water sports or activities, is the pump waterproof?

- How easy are the buttons to push? Delivering a bolus, for example, should be easy for the pump user, but accidentally giving a bolus should not be easy during careless gestures or around inquisitive friends.

- What level of customer service is provided by the manufacturer? 24-hour telephone support? Assistance with insurance coverage? Warranty? Trial period?

- In case of pump problems, do you have a backup pump? If not, how quickly can you get a replacement?

- What accessories come with the pump? Does the color of the pump matter?

- Do you need a delayed-delivery or square wave bolus for slow digestion, slow (low glycemic index) foods, or occasional brunches?

- How familiar is your diabetes team with the pump you want?

When selecting infusion sets (the part that actually goes under the skin), consider the following:

- How much subcutaneous (fat) tissue do you have?

- What infusion sites will you use?

- If you have never used the abdomen (preferred site) before for injections, will using it for the pump site be a problem?

- Are metal needles as comfortable for you as Teflon sets?

- Will you need a device to aid with insertion of the infusion set?

Pumps are often shipped with teflon infusion sets, but today's metal needles are very comfortable and may reduce the risk of delivery problems. Some lean adults and children may prefer today's very fine gauge 90-degree needles which come in a variety of lengths. Others will want the ability to use an insertion device like the Sof-Serter to place their catheter. Others will want a set like the Rapid that is easiest to apply. Some may also have a preference for where the infusion set disconnects.

We suggest that you try inserting different infusion sets to determine which is most comfortable and easiest to insert. Which has the features you desire? Occasionally, one set may cause skin sensitivity while another does not. An informed decision can avoid an investment in several boxes of infusion sets that may not be appropriate. It can also make or break the satisfaction you get out of pumping.

Examples

Here are some examples of people who wear pumps. They are motivated by a variety of circumstances, and experience different benefits from pumping.

Amy

Amy, a software engineer and racquet ball fanatic in her late 20's, has had diabetes for 12 years. During most of this time she has been plagued by repeated highs and lows, largely triggered by her sensitivity to insulin and her varied daily activities.

With an average total daily insulin dose of only 19 units, her blood sugar drops 120 mg/dl on each unit of insulin. Her sensitivity and low doses have made precise dosing very difficult despite four or more injections a day.

Amy began pumping after being found unconscious behind the wheel of her car in a shopping mall parking lot. Since starting on the pump, she marvels at the stability of her blood sugars, and her husband and coworkers are thrilled with her mellowed personality. "I feel like a regular person," she says.

George

George is in his 60's and retired after selling his plumbing business. He's had Type 2 diabetes for over 15 years. He was first treated with oral agents for 10 years, then switched to injections when three oral agents could no longer lower his morning blood sugars. Even on metformin, glyburide, and nearly 100 units of insulin a day, his fasting readings continued to stay above 150 mg/dl. After considering a pump for two years, he finally agreed to try it at his wife's insistence. Three months later, George says, "Now I don't have to work so hard to have a good day, and I wake up in the morning with normal readings. I use half as much insulin, and my triglyceride levels are normal."

Frank

Frank, a tile layer with Type 1 diabetes for 37 years, has experienced progressive nerve damage symptoms for the last ten years, first tingling in his feet that turned to numbness climbing his legs. He finally admitted to making up most of his blood sugar records. He started taking his testing and control seriously when he began having trouble getting to sleep because of shooting pains in his legs that got worse near bedtime, only mildly relieved by medication taken at that time. After ten months on his pump with doses adjusted to match real blood sugar readings, Frank sleeps normally with no need for neuropathy medication. "The feeling in my feet is definitely better," he admits.

Are You Ready For Pumping?

1. Are you motivated to control your blood sugars?

    not very 0   1   2   3   4   5 very   _____

2. How many blood sugar tests do you do each day?

    0   1   2   3   4   5   _____

3 Number of injections per day:

    0   1   2   3   4   5   _____

4. Do you record your test results?

    yes (5pts)   no (0 pts)   _____

5. Do you adjust your insulin from test results?

    yes (5pts)   no (0 pts)   _____

6. Do you adjust insulin for carb content of meals?*

    yes (5pts)   no (0 pts)   _____

7. Do you adjust insulin to bring down occ. highs?*

    yes (5pts)   no (0 pts)   _____

8. Do you adjust L/N/UL as needed for exercise, etc?*

    yes (5pts)   no (0 pts)   _____

9. Do you get regular HbA1c tests to validate control?

    yes (5pts)   no (0 pts)   _____

10. Do you call your physician when problems occur?

    yes (5pts)   no (0 pts)   _____

    Total   _____

* Seek your physician's help on any insulin adjustment until he or she is confidant you can make your own adjustments.

Your Pump Eligibility Scorecard

Score	What it means:
0-9	Who's in charge?
10-19	Honesty does pay.
20-29	Can you improve somewhere?
30-39	Just minor changes needed.
40-50	When do you start?

Tips For Better Control

• Insulin reactions and unexpected highs are less likely if you test your blood sugars often.

• "Brittle" diabetes is just an easy name for incorrect dosing or variable insulin action. This instability occurs only when insulin is being given in the wrong amount or at the wrong time.

• If your basals and boluses are correctly set, it will be easier to keep your blood sugars stable and in the normal range most of the time.

• To correct patterns of highs and lows, understand the timing of your insulin and its potency in relation to food and exercise.

• Living a varied lifestyle with fixed meal boluses and basal rates spells disaster. For a free lifestyle, you must learn to adjust your basals and boluses to match your changing lifestyle.

• Life changes. Everyone needs to adjust their basals and boluses occasionally.

• Know when to contact your physician, and don't hesitate to do so. Your physician's job is to help you keep yourself healthy.

• Be involved in your control. It is, after all is said, your life.

Don't think! Thinking is the enemy of creativity. It's self-conscious, and anything self-conscious is lousy. You can't try to do things; you simply must do them.

Ray Bradbury

CHAPTER 5

What Do You Need To Start?

Pump training can help you succeed. A comprehensive pump training program will likely include pump operation, lifestyle issues, control factors, and backup resources. Many of these will be covered in detail in later chapters.

We recommend that you read this book in its entirety prior to your first day on your pump. Read and review the first 12 chapters, in particular, for success on start-up. These chapters also make a great reference if any problems arise later.

Mastering the following skills before starting will be richly rewarded:

Basic Pump Operation

- How to insert batteries
- How to program basal rates
- How to give boluses
- How to place the reservoir into the pump
- How to attach the infusion set to the reservoir
- How to prepare the insertion site
- How to insert the needle or catheter
- How to identify the alarms
- How to stop or suspend the pump
- How to review pump memory for current basal rates and for previous boluses or alarms
- Where to obtain pump supplies

Lifestyle Issues

- How to set up the pump and insert the infusion set
- Daily pump routines
- How to wear the pump
- How to handle school, friends, family
- How to take a pump vacation
- How to avoid weight gain

Control Factors to Know

- The timing and action of the insulin you use
- What the basal rates and boluses are designed to do
- How to count carbohydrates in food
- How to test basal rates
- How to test carb boluses and high blood sugar boluses
- When to use temporary basal rates or square wave boluses
- How to chart blood sugars, carbs, basals and boluses, etc.
- How to analyze blood sugar patterns
- What to do to correct unwanted patterns
- How to handle highs on the pump
- How to handle lows on the pump

Backup Resources

- 24-hour phone numbers for your manufacturer and your health care team
- Who to contact if problems with the pump or blood sugar control occur

Supply List

- Insulin: Lilly Humalog™ (lyspro), Novo-Nordisk Novolog™ (release expected soon), Novo-Nordisk Velosulin™ Regular, or standard Regular insulin
- Reservoir or syringe: Specific to each pump
- Infusion set: teflon and metal needle sets are available, with some pictured on the next page.
- Disinfectant for infusion site: 3M IV Prep™, Betadine™ Solution, or Hibiclens™
- Adhesive material: 3M IV 3000™, Johnson & Johnson Bio-occlusive Material, High Performance Tegaderm™, Polyskin™, or Opsite™
- Tapes for safety loop: silk tape, 3M Micropore™ tape, Smith and Nephew Hypafix™

Table 5.1 A Wide Variety Of Infusion Sets To Choose From

	Name(s)	Infusor Type	Infusor Base	Detachable?
	Disetronic *Classic*™ MiniMed *Polyfin QR Bent Needle*™ Pureline *Basic*™	Metal 27 guage 30 degree insertion	Plain needle or Cotton	QR, Yes Others, No
	Disetronic *Rapid*™ Pureline *Contact*™	Metal 8, 10, 12 mm 90 degree insertion	Cotton	No
	MiniMed *Sof-set Ultimate QR*™ MiniMed *Sof-set Micro QR*™	Teflon 6, 8,10,12 mm 90 degree insertion	Plastic	Yes
	Disetronic *Ultraflex Soft*™	Teflon 8, 10, 12 mm 90 degree insertion	Cotton	Yes
	Disetronic *Tender*™ MiniMed *Silhouette*™ PureLine *Comfort*™	Teflon 30-45 degree insertion	Cotton	Yes
	Disetronic *Diaport*™, now in clinical trials	Surgically implanted under the skin with tube into peritoneal cavity	Port at skin	Yes, at port

- Skin Prep™ is a useful skin preparation for those with allergies to tape

- To reduce loss of insertion set from perspiration, use an odorless antiperspirant (not a deodorant) spray, Skin Tac H™, Applicare's Compound Benzoin Swabstick™, or Drysol™.

- Blood sugar testing equipment: meter, strips, lancets, lancing device, charts, charting software

- Low blood sugar treatment: glucagon injection kit (prescription), glucose tablets or dextrose candy, Monojel™

Your training should include ample time for questions, answers, and practice with your pump, usually a total of 3 to 6 hours. Most pumps are started in outpatient settings such as medical offices or clinics. With careful monitoring and close telephone contact, this approach works very well, and allows basal rates and boluses to be individualized to normal daily routines. Some physicians prefer to hospitalize new pumpers for a few days to establish and evaluate the pump program.

With either approach, you can speed up your training by reviewing the training materials provided in this book, as well as those from your diabetes center and the pump manufacturer. Watch the manufacturer's videotape at least twice, and carefully read the owner's manual. Try to gain as much experience as possible with your pump by pushing its buttons to set basal rates, give boluses, and review memory before actually starting on it. Of course, if you do not have access to the pump before starting on it, this practice manipulation of the pump may have to be skipped.

Regardless of where you start on a pump, you'll need 24-hour telephone access to your physician/health provider team, and to your insulin pump manufacturer to deal with any unanticipated problems.

Record Keeping

Although you may not look forward to keeping records, they provide the critical information needed to quickly solve problems when your control is not what you would like. They also help you spot new problems so that control can be maintained. To accurately test basal rates and boluses and to avoid dangerous low blood sugars, you will need to record basal rates and all

When To Test And Record:

- Before and after each meal and at bedtime, and at 2 a.m. on at least 3 of the first 7 nights.

- Any time you think your blood sugar may be low or high.

- Before driving, and during trips that last more than an hour.

- When drinking alcohol.

Record your blood sugar tests, food choices, carb counts, and activity in the *Smart Charts*, and bring your charts to all clinic visits.

boluses, blood sugar readings, total carbs eaten and the time they are eaten, times of suspected lows, carbs eaten to treat lows, as well as any extra exercise or activity. Recording this information is especially important prior to and at the time you start on a pump, as it speeds the determination of correct basals and boluses.

It's important to keep good records at all times, but especially at any time you have a problem with blood sugar control. Charting is covered in Chapter 6. Some of today's blood sugar meters also offer advanced recording and analysis options.

Which Insulin Do You Use?

Pumps do not use any long-acting insulin but only a short-acting, clear insulin. Although it has not been FDA-approved for use in the pump, Humalog is almost universally preferred over Regular by researchers, clinicians, and pumpers. Since Humalog became available in 1996, many studies researching its safety and effectiveness in the pump have been conducted and reported at American Diabetes Association annual conventions and in major diabetes journals.[39, 40, 41, 42]

A general survey of clinicians and pump users suggests that about 90% of pump users currently use Humalog in their pump. Humalog is undergoing the FDA review process at this time, and is expected to be approved for pump use. Your physician/ health care team will guide you toward an appropriate insulin to use.

Humalog is generally preferred over Regular because its quick action time is close to the way natural insulin works. Following an injection or bolus, Humalog starts to work in 10 minutes, peaks at 1.5 hours and is gone by 3.5 hours, providing more precise insulin delivery and faster response times.

Because Humalog is fast-acting, it offers users more flexibility and control. One of the major ways it does this is by matching food digestion time better than Regular does. When you use Humalog, you can take carbohydrate boluses whenever you decide to eat. This means you can choose to eat or not eat, as the occasion arises. The simple procedure of taking Humalog with your first bite prevents severe lows related to delayed eating. This is especially good for people with Type I diabetes who experience hypoglycemia unawareness.

Food digestion generally matches Humalog's action. Although foods vary in their speed of digestion, as measured by the glycemic index, most will begin to digest about 10 minutes after eating, peak in the blood in about 30 to 60 minutes, and no longer have an effect after 2.5 or 3 hours. Humalog's action parallels the typical digestion of food which allows the post-meal blood sugar to stay well-controlled. Post-meal spiking is reduced and Humalog does not continue working after the meal is gone. For the occasional situation where food digestion is slow, pumps can be programmed in a number of ways to allow Humalog to accommodate to these situations.

Humalog's fast action time allows you to lower high blood sugars faster and match exercise better by adjusting basals and boluses with less lead time. The shorter, more precise action time means that unused insulin doesn't accumulate in the body through the day and increase your risk of nighttime lows and, over time, daytime lows.

A person using Humalog in the pump may need less insulin than when Regular is used because meals are covered more precisely and high blood sugars are lowered more quickly. Although no research has indicated this conclusively, it may be better for your body to attain blood sugar control with lower levels of insulin.

When you use Humalog, determining the cause for both lows and highs becomes easier. If afternoon lows are occurring on a pump with Humalog, only the lunch bolus or the basal insulin can be at fault. To find out which is the culprit, simply skip lunch

---

Tips For Using Humalog

- Use fast carbs, such as glucose tablets, for all lows

- Don't skip or delay a meal once you've bolused (unless lowering a high blood sugar)

- Be careful using Humalog with low glycemic index foods to avoid early lows and late highs.

- You don't need to overtreat an insulin reaction that happens 3 or 4 hours after a Humalog bolus--- most of Humalog's effect is gone by then.

- Avoid using a pump's suspend feature for exercise or low blood sugars. With complete suspension, Humalog levels drop rapidly over 60 to 90 minutes, which is then followed by a rapid rise in blood sugar.

- **Be safe, not sorry.** Take Humalog by injection at the **FIRST** high blood sugar reading over 300 mg/dl (17 mmol). If any delivery problem occurs with Humalog in your pump, blood sugars can begin to rise as early as 60 to 80 minutes later, and ketoacidosis could start within 3 to 5 hours.

one day and skip the bolus of Humalog ordinarily taken to cover it. If the blood sugar drops in this situation, too much basal insulin is responsible. But if the blood sugar stays flat or varies by only 30 points when lunch is skipped, the basal is correct and the lunch Humalog has to be the culprit.

You will find that Humalog presents specific challenges. Do not delay a meal after giving a Humalog carb bolus when your blood sugar is normal. The most common cause for severe low blood sugars is delaying a meal, or becoming distracted and not eating at all. Because a blood sugar drop will start faster and fall faster on Humalog, any delay in eating after bolusing can become critical quickly.

Although covering high glycemic index foods, such as cold breakfast cereal or a scone, is not as great a concern, a problem may arise with slower carbs, those lower on the glycemic index. Meals like pasta al dente or a bean burrito may raise the blood sugar too slowly for Humalog. Eating foods that convert slowly to glucose can cause the blood sugar to go low at one or two hours after eating but then rise after the Humalog is gone. Some dinner meals may now cause high blood sugars before breakfast the following morning if the only bolus is the one given at the time of eating.

For people who have slow digestion due to gastroparesis, a fast insulin may not always be preferred. Fortunately, even with a fast insulin like Humalog, a pump can be programmed to match the delayed digestion found with gastroparesis. Smaller boluses can be combined with a larger daytime basal delivery, or a temporary basal rate increase can be used to cover food over a longer period of time, rather than rely on a large carb bolus. A "square wave" bolus, which is delivered over a long, rectangular period of time, is another alternative. Discuss these options with your physician.

Select The Infusion Site

The abdomen is a convenient place to insert the infusion set. Variations in insulin absorption that once were created when different sites were used for infusion of Regular insulin[43,44] largely disappear with the use of Humalog. Any site above or below the belt line which is "pinchable" can be chosen.

Infusion sites are rotated to prevent scarring, which can interfere with insulin absorption. In the abdominal area, the infusion set can be placed anywhere from just below the rib cage to just above the pubic area, to within two fingerwidths of the belly button extending to the sides, basically anywhere you can "pinch an inch". In the buttocks, the area near the pocket line works well because you do not sit or sleep on it. The front and sides of the thighs work well for those who don't wear tight pants. The outer side of the biceps is generally preferred for the arms.

Four or more infusion sites are preferred for rotation purposes. Sites can be rotated by area, i.e., right upper quadrant, right lower quadrant, left lower quadrant, left upper quadrant. Site rotation can also be done in small steps, i.e., move the new site about 2 inches across the abdomen from the last one.

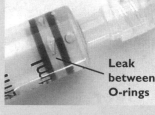
A convenient way to remember your rotation schedule is to pick two days of the
week to change your infusion site and always use these two days. For instance, always
change on Sundays and Wednesdays.

Prepare The Reservoir And Infusion Set

1. Fill the reservoir with insulin after following the O-ring procedure described
in the box above.

2. Get rid of air bubbles in the reservoir by holding the reservoir in the palm of
your hand and pointing the needle up with the air bubble toward you. Tip the reservoir so the bottom or plunger end is slightly farther away than the needle end. Flick
the reservoir with a fingernail or pen until the air bubble enters the neck of the
reservoir. Then squirt insulin into the insulin bottle to get rid of the air bubble.

Little champagne bubbles are harder to get rid of,
but they are harmless. Larger bubbles can displace a
significant amount of insulin and should be eliminated.
If air bubbles are seen in the infusion line, an inch of air
in the line is equal to half a unit of insulin. In most
cases, up to an inch of air in the line is not of concern.

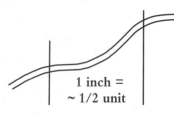

1 inch = ~ 1/2 unit

3. Detach the needle from the reservoir and
immediately replace it with the hub on the infusion set.
When tightening, grip the reservoir at the hub. To avoid hub leaks, be sure that the
connection between the infusion set and the reservoir has been firmly tightened.

4. Prime or fill the infusion line with insulin before insertion until a droplet forms at the end of the line. Some pump reservoirs are easier to prime before inserting them into the pump, while others can be conveniently primed by the pump itself.

5. Look closely for any sign of an insulin leak between the O-rings, as shown on the previous page. Replace the reservoir if any liquid, mist or bubbles are noted. Even seemingly small leaks in this location can cause a rapid loss of control.

6. Place the reservoir in the pump. Recheck the O-rings and then give 2 unit boluses until insulin can be seen exiting from the tip of the infusion set.

7. You are now ready to prepare the site and insert the infusion set.

Prepare Your Site

Use the sterile technique described here while setting up your pump and infusion site. This will help prevent serious infections, such as abscesses or an infection that requires surgical drainage. Common sources for bacteria include the hands, the breath, and the skin at the infusion site, plus any contact the infusion set might have with counter tops, etc.

1. To reduce the bacteria count, wash your hands with soap and water. Avoid touching the reservoir needle, the tip of the reservoir, the end of the infusion set, or the top of the insulin bottle.

2. Whenever close viewing is needed, hold your reservoir or infusion set at eye level above your nose. Many germs reside in the nose and breath coming out of the nose. Don't breathe or blow directly on the pump, the reservoir, the infusion set or the infusion site, as this may lead to a site infection. If you have had a history of minor skin infections in the past, you may want to obtain a surgical mask to wear over your nose and mouth during setup to decrease the risk for infections.

3. Scrub the infusion site on the skin with an antiseptic solution. Use IV Prep pads, 1% or 2% iodine (Betadine™ Solution), or chlorhexidine (Hibiclens™) to cleanse a site two inches in diameter on the skin.

4. When the site is dry, place a bio-occlusive adhesive like 3M IV Prep or Johnson & Johnson's Bio-occlusive Material over this area. These materials as well as others like Tegaderm™ or Polyskin™ reduce site irritation.

Practice Sterile Technique

1. Wash your hands well.

2. Do not breathe or blow on your equipment or infusion site.

3. Do not touch your face or nose.

4. Eliminate bacteria from the skin where you plan to place the infusion set with IV Prep, Hibiclens, or betadine.

5. Place a bioocclusive material like IV 3000™ or J&J Bio-occlusive Material onto the prepared skin so the infusion set can be placed through this.

Is Your Insulin OK?

Anytime you have unexplained high blood sugars, check your insulin. To visually check Humalog or Regular, grasp the bottle by the neck and turn it upside down. Bubbles will always rise, but clumps of insulin, sometimes very small, will fall or can be seen attached to the inside wall of the bottle. If you see any, your insulin has gone bad. Bad insulin may also have a slightly yellow or brown color to it. Good insulin will appear as clear as water.

Insulin is more likely to go bad in a pump reservoir than a bottle. If there is any question of potency, always replace your reservoir and infusion set as soon as unexpected high blood sugars occur. Inject insulin with a syringe to ensure the high blood sugar is corrected. Use a fresh bottle with a different lot number, even if you need to make an extra trip to your pharmacy.

Humalog insulin, in particular, should be kept refrigerated at 36 to 45 degrees Fahrenheit until just prior to use, when it can be warmed to room temperature. Cold insulin may form champagne bubbles over several hours after being placed in the reservoir, but this is a minor problem.

Insulin goes bad when exposed to sunlight, heat, cold, or agitation. Exposure to temperature extremes may occur during transit to a distributor, to your pharmacy, or to your home. It becomes apparent only after unexpected highs. **Do not assume all highs are your fault.** Chapter 22 covers some of the problems, besides bad insulin, that can cause a rapid loss of control.

Insert The Infusion Set

1. Insert the infusion set into the skin through the bio-occlusive adhesive. If using a needle, position the metal needle so it is parallel to your beltline but not underneath it. Teflon sets contain dead space in them after insertion. A bolus of 0.8 unit to 1.0 unit is needed for the Comfort™, Silhouette™ or Tender™, and 0.5 unit for Sof-Sets™ to fill this dead space after a teflon infusion set is inserted. Have a qualified instructor demonstrate how to properly insert these sets.

2. Once the infusion set is inserted and secured in place, loop the infusion line a short distance away and tape this loop against the skin with a piece of Micropore™ tape or other adhesive. This safety loop can be placed about an inch away from the infusion site and prevents the infusion set from being dislodged should the infusion line be accidentally pulled.

3. Change the infusion site at least every 72 hours to prevent skin irritation or infection or an abscess that may require an antibiotic or surgery.

4. Check the infusion site daily or whenever you suspect redness, swelling or bleeding. Change the infusion site immediately if any of these occur.

5. Be sure to inspect your infusion site for problems if your blood sugars are high.

Sweating from heat or exercise can cause the infusion set to come loose. If this is a problem, use a plain unscented antiperspirant (not deodorant) on the skin to reduce sweating.

Avoid Infections

If redness or inflammation occurs at a site, assume the worst. Immediately change to a new infusion site using a new infusion set. Call your physician immediately if the inflamed site is larger than a dime. A topical antibiotic cream used early may slow an infection when one is just starting.

If you have an infection, give insulin by injection until an oral antibiotic has been started and the site clears. Do not use the inflamed site again until the inflammation and swelling have totally cleared. You may not even want to use your pump until an antibiotic has been started, as an infection can spread to a new site.

Nonfatal toxic shock has been reported from infusion site infections. One case was reported in an unwilling teenager, and another was in a pumper who followed instructions that used only alcohol as a disinfectant and allowed several days pass between infusion site changes.[45] Always treat site infections with the utmost care. If you are prone to skin infections, you may want to discuss with your physician having a broad spectrum antibiotic on hand for early treatment of a site infection. Fungal infections following prolonged use of a site have also been reported.

Sterile technique and hygiene are your best insurance against infections.[46] To prevent infections, follow the steps in "Prepare Your Site" on page 39.

What Follow-up Will You Need?

After you go on a pump, close follow-up is essential for success. Easy access to your health provider helps sort out problems quickly and is especially important during the first week or two after starting the pump. When you run into a pump problem, communicate it clearly and accurately. Tell your health provider why you're calling and why you believe this problem is occurring. Have all your charting information close at hand to give quick information on blood sugars, time of day, carb intake, and activity levels.

Reduce Insertion Pain

Some people feel pain and discomfort when inserting needles or catheters. Luckily, there are ways to numb the skin to make needle insertion more comfortable. Emla™ cream, a numbing cream available at pharmacies, can be applied to the skin about an hour before insertion. Another easy alternative is to place an ice cube on the site right before insertion to trick the nerve endings into feeling cold instead of pain. It's a handy alternative for children and adults with a needle phobia. Many people find these aids unnecessary after the first few weeks or months of pump use.

Be sure you understand any instructions you are given--dates of follow-up appointments, what to bring, and who to call for various kinds of information during the process. Keep all the follow-up appointments you are given.

For follow-up:

- Get a phone number for 24-hour medical contact. Know who and when to call for information or help, such as during extremely high or low blood sugars, site problems (itching, infection), and emergencies.

- Remember that your starting basals and boluses are only estimates. An insulin adjustment, usually a small reduction in your doses, may be needed within the first 2 or 3 days, with another reduction a few days later.

- Symptoms for insulin reactions may not be as noticeable on a pump due to the more gradual drop in blood sugars. Check your blood sugar more often than you did on injections to avoid this.

- Know when to arrange phone follow-up: after how many days, with what test results, or as needed, such as for blood sugars over 250 mg/dl (13.9 mmol) on 2 consecutive readings or less than 50 mg/dl (2.8 mmol) at any time.

- Arrange follow-up appointments as requested, for instance in 1, 3, and 6 weeks.

- Fill out your *Smart Charts* and take them to every clinic visit so your care provider can quickly evaluate your blood sugar patterns, boluses, carb intake, etc.

- Contact your pump company for any technical problems (alarms, unclear messages, etc.) with the pump. A 24-hour contact number is on the back of each pump.

- If you have any eye damage, arrange follow-up with your ophthalmologist. Rapidly improved control on a pump can temporarily worsen existing retinopathy.

Tips On Pumping

High Blood Sugars: High blood sugars can be a very serious problem. Any time your blood sugar readings are over 250 mg/dl (13.9 mmol) twice in a row without a good reason, take an injection to lower your blood sugar and replace your syringe and infusion set immediately, using a new bottle of insulin. Check your blood ketone level with a specialized meter like the Precision Xtra™, or your urine with Ketostix™ for ketones. Call your physician/health care team immediately if ketones are over 0.6 mmol/L in the blood or at moderate or large levels in the urine. Test your blood sugar at 30 minute intervals to make sure you are correcting the problem.

HbA1c Tests: Check your HbA1c levels every three to six months to assist in evaluating your overall blood sugar control. Remember that the HbA1c test cannot detect erratic blood sugars nor replace frequent home monitoring. Its purpose is to provide an average of the last several weeks' blood sugar readings[40] and is most reflective of the last four to six weeks' blood sugars.

Lifestyle Issues

Showers and bathing

With detachable infusion sets, simply disconnect the infusion line from the infusion set. Reattach after the bath or shower (30-45 min.). Always leave the pump in run mode as this reduces your chance of a clog and keeps you from forgetting to restart a suspended pump.

If you are not using a detachable set and if your pump is waterproof, simply hang the infusion set around your neck with the pump at the end in a bag, use a Shower-Allower which has suction cups that attach to the shower wall, or place the pump in a shower organizer, or on the side of the tub. As an extra precaution, the pump can be placed in a plastic bag or in a velcro camping bag to keep it dry.

Sleeping

Place the pump free on the bed, under a pillow, in a pajama pocket, or clamped to shorts or a soft belt. Unique Pump Accessories and pump manufacturers offer a wide variety of clothing and cases like the Sleep-T, Flannel Boxers, or a Waist-It that make wearing the pump easier and more comfortable.

Sex

If you and your partner are comfortable with the pump, let the pump take care of itself in a convenient location. Women may want to attach the pump to a garter belt with the pump's belt clip. With detachable infusion sets, simply detach the pump. You can remain off the pump 60 minutes with Humalog or 90 minutes with Regular, but staying detached longer will cause blood sugars to rise. Ketoacidosis can develop if you stay off for four hours or more. Be sure to reattach your pump before falling asleep.

Hot Tubs and Saunas

Heat can make proteins like insulin harden. The heat found in most saunas and some hot tubs can turn an enjoyable experience into high blood sugars and ketoacidosis. If your infusion set disconnects, disconnect before entering. If your set does not detach, remove the whole apparatus while in a hot tub or sauna and use a new set afterward. Recent research has shown that using a hot tub can lower blood sugars, so watch your blood sugar carefully during and afterward.

Removing Reservoir: Do not remove a reservoir from a pump unless you are changing the set. Never prime an infusion set, nor attempt to free a clogged infusion line while you still have the infusion set in place. You risk accidentally injecting yourself with large doses of insulin.

Diluting Insulin: People on small daily doses often have more variable blood sugars because of their sensitivity to insulin. Today's DC motors and frequent insulin delivery allow most pumpers on small daily doses to use full-strength insulin. Diluting insulin can be considered to improve dosing accuracy. Diluting may occasionally help those taking less than 20 to 25 total units a day, or those using a basal rate of 0.4 units or less per hour.

Luckily, insulin can be diluted with a diluent from the manufacturer. The diluent for NPH insulin is clear and can be used with Humalog insulin as long as it is used within 14 days of mixing. Velosulin diluent appears to last longer after mixing with Humalog and may be obtained from Novo Nordisk by special request. Insulin mixed 1 to 1 with diluent is easy to work with.

With a 1 to 1 dilution, if you keep the same basal rate on the pump, the actual insulin delivered by the pump is half of the amount shown on the pump. That is, a basal rate of 0.7 u/hr would now be delivering only 0.35 u/hr, and a bolus of 5.0 units of diluted insulin would deliver 2.5 units of actual insulin. Some pumps can also be set for U-50 insulin delivery which lets the pump read 2.5 units when 2.5 units of diluted insulin is delivered.

Although dilution is inconvenient and must be precisely carried out, the inconvenience of dilution can be quickly offset if blood sugar control improves and the risk for low blood sugars is decreased from more exact insulin delivery.[47]

Ketoacidosis: Whenever insulin flow is interrupted by a leak, clog, displaced infusion set, or removal of the pump, ketoacidosis may begin in about 4 hours with Humalog, or after about 5 hours with Regular. Ketoacidosis can be dangerous especially if it occurs at night, as can happen if an infusion set becomes displaced at bedtime.

Change insulin reservoirs and/or infusion sets before the evening hours, preferably in the morning. This allows normal daytime testing to quickly pick up any serious problem with insulin delivery due to a set or pump problem. If you must change an infusion set at night, set an alarm for three hours after your set change and check your blood sugar at that time.

Severe high blood sugars and ketoacidosis can be very serious medical problems. These life-threatening conditions are most often seen in Type 1 or insulin-dependent diabetes because the body does not produce its own insulin.

Ketoacidosis also can be triggered by bad insulin, a severe infection, or a serious illness. Additionally, it can be triggered in Type 1 or Type 2 diabetes by the stress of an illness like pneumonia or a heart attack. In children and adolescents with Type 1 diabetes, ketoacidosis can be triggered by normal growth spurts if basal rates and boluses have not been raised to meet this increasing need for insulin. Keep a meter like the Precision Xtra™ that can check for ketones in the blood as well as checking blood sugars, or Ketostix™ or Ketodiastix™ urine test strips handy for checking your urine for the presence of ketones. See Chapter 17 for more information on ketoacidosis.

A pump is only as good as the technique of the person using it. Dedicate yourself to learning and using excellent technique.

How To Take Pump Vacations

Occasionally you may want or need to discontinue pump use for a short period. There may be a pump problem, an infection at the infusion site, a day at the beach, contact sport activities, or sexual relations. Table 5.2 provides instructions on how to maintain control while off the pump for different lengths of time.

Table 5.2 Suggestions For Pump Vacations	
Time off pump	**Try this:**
Less than 1 hour	Nothing if BG is OK. Bolus if BG is high or carbs will be eaten.
1 to 3.5 hours	Take a bolus before disconnecting to cover 80% of the basal during the time off your pump. Cover carbs with an injection or reconnect and bolus.
3.5 to 5 hours daytime	Take an injection of Regular to cover the basal rate during the time off the pump.
over 5 hours daytime	Take a bolus for first 2 hours of basal insulin and, if needed, to cover breakfast. Then take an injection of NPH or Lente at breakfast to cover 1.2 X basal need during time off pump. Cover later carbs with Humalog injections.
over 3.5 hours nighttime	Take a bolus for first 2 hours of basal insulin. Then take an injection of NPH or Lente at bedtime to cover 1.5 X basal need during 8 hours of sleep.
These are only suggestions. Carefully discuss your own specific doses with your physician.	

People who claw their way to the top are not likely to find very much wrong with the system that enabled them to rise.

Arthur Schlesinger, Jr.

Instructions For Pump Start

1. If you are using Lantus, Lente, or NPH insulin, this insulin should not be taken on

   ____/____, the morning of your pump start.

   If you are using Ultralente/U insulin, this insulin should not be taken on the evening

   of ____/____, the day before your pump start.

2. After stopping your longer-acting insulin, Humalog must be taken frequently, usually every three hours, to manage your blood sugar until you start on your pump.

   You will need to take _____units of _____insulin every _____hours to keep your blood sugar from rising, plus any additional insulin needed for carbs or high blood sugars. Check your blood sugar at least every 2-3 hours until you start on your pump. Frequent testing will also be required in the first few days after starting

3. Take only _____units of _____ insulin before breakfast on the day of your pump start. Do not take NPH, Lente, Lantus, or Ultralente that morning.

4. Eat your usual breakfast.

5. Bring these with you for your pump start:
   - Your blood sugar meter plus extra test strips
   - Your logbook with blood sugar and diet records
   - Insulin for the pump: ❑ Humalog ❑ Velosulin ❑ Regular
   - Treatment for low blood sugars: glucose tablets, fruit, fruit juice, or candy
   - Food for lunch and snacks
   - Your pump
   - All pump supplies, including your pump user manual
   - _____
   - _____

6. Your appointment for Pump Training is scheduled for _____ am/pm on ____/____/____

   To change your appointment, please call ( ) _____--_____

Charting

Normal blood sugars come from insulin entering the bloodstream in the correct amount at the right time to balance the other factors that raise or lower the blood sugar. To get a complete picture of how all the factors are impacting your control, chart basal rates, boluses, carbs, activity, stress, and anything else important. This takes some time and effort, but it is always the best way to see how your insulin and carbs can be adjusted to bring your blood sugars under control.

This chapter describes

- Why charting is important
- How to chart
- A sample chart with analysis

Then in the chapters that follow, we'll show you how to use this information with your pump to gain better control.

Why Chart?

Life changes. Days lengthen and shorten, activity increases and decreases, week-ends differ from weekdays, stress rises and falls, food intake shifts from more carbs in the summer to more fat in the winter, and meals may be delayed or skipped. All of these affect how much insulin you need, as well as your blood sugar levels.

Better than traditional logbooks, charts

- Let you collect in one place everything affecting your control
- Provide a graphical format to show the rise and fall of your blood sugars

- Tell you whether your blood sugars are above or below your desired range
- Reveal the time of day problems typically occur
- Help you precisely pinpoint the source of control problems

Over time, charts tell you if you are getting where you want to go. They become your guide and let you know whether the changes you make are really helping you gain better control. Charts allow you to visualize the patterns in your readings so that you become aware of any consistent rise or fall of the blood sugars. Patterns may reveal frequent lows in the afternoon, consistently high readings in the morning, certain meals that cause your blood sugars to go high or low, or the effects of stress or a change in weight on your readings. As you gather information on your charts, these patterns become apparent to you and your health care team.

The discipline required in charting leads to freedom from the worry of unknown internal damage, freedom from the annoyance and frustration of test results that show blood sugars out of control, and freedom from the mood swings caused by high and low blood sugars. Most importantly, your charting gives you the freedom to eat, work and exercise the way you want.

Smart Charts are the record system recommended in this book. A blank *Smart Chart* is shown on the next page. *Smart Charts* are the record system part of *My Other CheckBook* and are a perfect size to slip into a checkbook cover for easy carrying in your pocket or purse.

What Do I Put On My Charts?

The more information you place on your charts, the easier it becomes to control your blood sugars. Charting reveals patterns and problems more quickly than even today's advanced meters. Keep your charts handy for quick access and easy record keeping. Recording the following information can help identify and correct unwanted blood sugar patterns and speed your path to good control. Many people use different colors or shapes on their *Smart Charts* to indicate different activities or events.

Activity

Record any physical activity, exercise or work that is greater than normal in the activity area at the top of the graph. For instance, if you golf only on Saturdays, record it. Infrequent activities like weekend golfing usually have to be balanced with extra carbohydrate or a reduction in insulin doses. On the other hand, if you run 5 miles at the same time each day, this is normal daily activity for you and probably requires no change in your usual daily routine once your basals and boluses are correctly adjusted for your run.

Rank your physical activity on a personal 1 to 5 scale. A "1" indicates a mild increase in activity, while you would give a "5" to activities that are strenuous. For instance, if sitting behind a desk is your usual work activity, but you spend the day

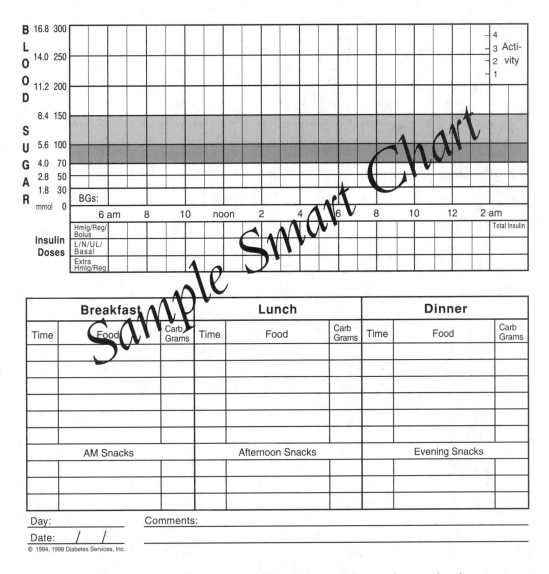

		Breakfast			Lunch			Dinner	
Time	Food	Carb Grams	Time	Food	Carb Grams	Time	Food	Carb Grams
	AM Snacks			Afternoon Snacks			Evening Snacks	

Day: _____ Comments: _____

Date: __ / __ / __ _____

moving your files and records to a new office, you would record a number between "1" and "5" during the appropriate workday hours, based on how much extra activity moving required.

If you began a running program and become quite winded during this new exercise, you would graph a "5" on your chart at the time of the run. After you run for a few days or weeks, this same run may no longer be strenuous for you and then would be listed as a "4" or a "3."

Also record activity that is less than normal, especially if it is a significant decline or goes on for several days. For instance, if you usually do aerobic exercise every day, but you skip it for a week when you strain your knee, record this less-than-normal activity.

Your goal in recording activity is to see whether it is affecting your control. If control problems are seen related to activity, adjustments can be made. For more precise estimates of the carbohydrate intake and insulin adjustments for exercise, see Chapters 18 and 19 on Excarbs.

See area A on Figure 6.1 for an example of how to chart physical activity. This shows someone who rode a bicycle for an hour and a half (level 5) in the morning, and then helped a neighbor load dirt into a trailer (level 4) for 45 minutes that afternoon.

Blood Sugar Readings

Graphing blood sugars reveals patterns that allow insulin doses to be adjusted correctly when blood sugars are not in control. At least 4 tests a day are needed to adjust insulin doses: before each meal and at bedtime. Additional information can be gained by testing 1 or 2 hours after meals. A complete picture of blood sugar patterns requires seven tests a day. Occasionally, a test at 2 a.m. is also needed.

Also test whenever low blood sugar symptoms occur, unless the symptoms are severe enough that waiting to test would be dangerous. If severe symptoms occur, eat first and then test as soon as you can or ask someone else to test for you. It's important to check your blood sugar if you feel low. Other conditions, such as excitement, fatigue, stress, or anxiety can mimic the symptoms of a low blood sugar. Knowing how low your blood sugar is at the time lets you make precise corrections.

Continuous monitoring devices, like blood sugar meters, have enough internal memory to download tons of blood sugar data to a computer. However, writing these blood sugars down each time as they appear enables you to quickly spot trends and avoid highs and lows. Discuss with your physician how often to record your blood sugars manually, and in what circumstances you want to respond with a bolus or carb intake. A graph is a perfect place to plot your readings to see trends, and it also allows you to refer back to them whenever you find yourself in similar circumstances. Of course, you won't need to record every reading, so decide on a reasonable frequency for plotting your results.

Record every insulin reaction on your charts, regardless of whether a blood sugar test was done. Indicate all verified and suspected insulin reactions on the chart with a circle or an arrow, with size or color showing the severity of the reaction. For instance, if symptoms are mild, use a small circle or arrow. If severe, use a large circle or arrow. The first step for improving control is to eliminate severe and frequent insulin reactions. Identifying patterns allows insulin doses to be correctly adjusted. If you are using a continuous monitor, it's internal alarms help avoid severe lows, and quick pattern recognition lets basals and boluses be quickly adjusted to avoid most insulin reactions.

Area B in Figure 6.1 shows the areas where blood sugars can be graphed. Insulin reactions are noted at the bottom as circled blood sugars with lows at 10:30 a.m. and 5:30 p.m.

Basals and Boluses

On the lines in the middle of your chart, record your basal rates and the time and size of all boluses you give. Lines are provided for carbohydrate boluses, basal rate(s), and any high blood sugar boluses that are needed.

Basal rates don't need to be recorded every day, but record them every week or so and when they are change. How to adjust basals and boluses is covered in Chapters 10 to 13. Carefully record the size and timing of any boluses given to cover carbs, and record as well all extra insulin given to lower high blood sugars. High blood sugar boluses are discussed in Chapter 12.

Area C in Figure 6.1 shows a sample of one day's insulin doses.

Foods and Carb Counts

Counting carbs is the best way to measure and track the part of the food that raises your blood sugar. Counting carbs directly from a label, calculating them by weighing your food on a gram scale, or looking them up in a book are all relatively easy to do. See Chapter 7 to learn how to count carbs.

Record all the foods you eat and the number of carbs in them at the bottom of the chart. This lets you cover your carbs consistently and pick up unexpected blood sugar responses that may be tied to particular foods. By listing what you eat and its carb content, you can determine the effect these foods are having on your blood sugars. You will find some foods have undesirable effects while others thought to be "bad" may be perfectly fine.

Be as specific as you can. A general word like "cereal" won't do, as all cereals are not equal. Cheerios®, Grape Nuts®, Cornflakes®, and oatmeal have very different effects on blood sugars. "Sandwich" can have very different effects when comparing "sandwich: whole wheat/tuna/mayo, 32 grams" to "sandwich: ice cream, 68 grams."

Don't overlook what you eat to correct low blood sugars. If you don't record the 4 full graham crackers (44 grams) and 16 ounces of milk (24 grams) that you took for a nighttime reaction, you won't be able to determine why your blood sugar was 307 mg/dl the following morning.

List all foods, not just carbs. You may discover that foods with only a little carb in them, like cheese or nuts, have a subtle effect and cause your blood sugar to climb gradually for several hours after you eat them. It helps if you also estimate how much of these non-carb foods you've eaten. Estimate the amounts, like 2 ounces of cheese or 10 ounces of prime rib, on your charts.

A dietician can provide you with precise recommendations for your daily carb need as well as information on ways to improve your blood sugars and health through your food choices. The way to determine the ratio of Humalog or Regular to grams of carbohydrate is covered in Chapter 11.

Area D in Figure 6.1 shows list of food eaten and its carbohydrate content.

Emotions, Stress, Comments

In the comments section at the bottom of the Smart Chart page you can record any other information you feel is relevant. Items like weight change, which affect your insulin need, can be recorded. Emotions, stress and illness can all impact your blood sugars. This information might be "I have a cold," or "I woke up with a headache, may have had a reaction during the night." A high blood sugar before dinner might be explained by a comment that "work was very stressful today".

Emotions and blood sugars are a two-way street. Understanding their relationship can help in your blood sugar control. The brain controls the secretion of various stress hormones that interfere with insulin. The brain, however, depends entirely on blood sugar for fuel. When either high or low levels of sugar reach the brain, the response can be loss of memory, anger, irritability, slowed thinking, or depression.

When blood sugars rise, hormones that prevent depression are lowered. When depressed, a person has less energy to do the things needed for good control: thought-

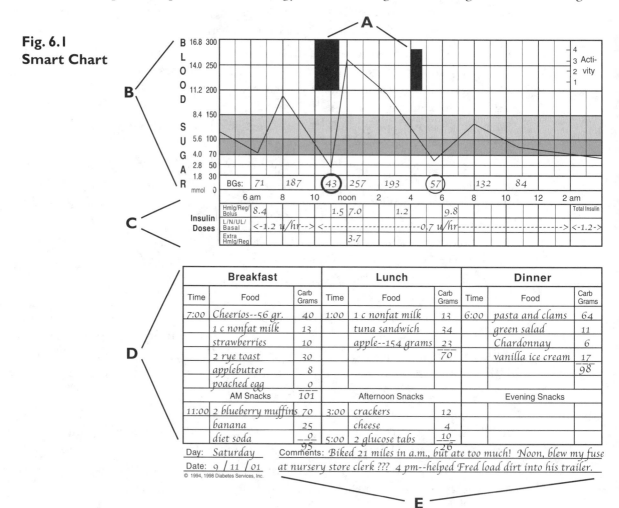

Fig. 6.1 Smart Chart

ful selection of foods, regular exercise, and rest. This can become a vicious cycle that needs to be broken.

The Comments section is the place to begin connecting your own emotions and blood sugars. Area E in Figure 6.1 shows an example.

Spot Your Blood Sugar Patterns

On a regular schedule, preferably once each week, review your completed charts for patterns of high and low blood sugars. For instance, every Saturday morning review the last seven days' charts. With a continuous monitor, you can pick up patterns after only a few days, allowing rapid basal and bolus testing as outlined in the next few chapters. Discuss how to adjust basals first and then boluses with your physician and health care team to correct unwanted patterns.

Look for any patterns in the following:

- Insulin reactions
- High blood sugars
- High blood sugars that follow insulin reactions
- Low blood sugars that follow highs
- High or low blood sugars that follow particular foods
- Drops in your blood sugars after exercise
- Differences between weekend and workday blood sugars

Show your charts to others, and listen to their suggestions. Another person, especially someone trained in diabetes care and focused on glucose control, will often see things that you miss. Diabetes personnel, in particular, understand the complexities of diabetes in daily life. If you have any uncertainty about a potential pattern or the need to adjust your insulin, be sure to contact your physician/health care team for advice. Use the knowledge and experience of others to simplify your path toward normal readings.

How long should you record in this detailed way? Data collected in your *Smart Charts* may be more extensive than normally needed. But when you start on a pump, charting the factors that influence your blood sugars allows you to understand and change them. After successfully stabilizing your blood sugars with your pump, you may only need a simple daily log. But if you go through a period when your control worsens, go back to the *Smart Charts* to help you regain control. Some people use *Smart Charts* all the time to help them maintain good eating habits and constantly stay on top of patterns in their blood sugars. Regular recording is a great habit for optimum pump results.

Sample Chart

On the next page is one day's chart for Sam, a pumper. Examine his chart carefully. Make your own decisions about what you would change if you were Sam and this were your chart. What is happening to his blood sugars? Are they out of the normal range? Why? What would you do about it? You may want to write your suggestions down on paper for ways to improve his blood sugars. After giving Sam's chart some thought about changes you would make, look at the analysis that follows for confirmation of your thinking. Don't peek!

Background

Sam has been using an insulin pump for 7 months. He weighs 161 pounds and leads an active lifestyle. He eats 2200 calories a day, with 1100 of these calories coming from carbohydrates. Most days he eats 275 grams of carbohydrate, with 80 grams for breakfast, 95 for lunch and afternoon snack, and 100 for dinner, although this and his meal boluses vary.

Sam's total daily insulin dose (basals plus boluses) averages 50 units a day. From previous testing (Chapter 11) Sam knows he needs one unit of Humalog for each 10 grams of carbohydrate in his meals. When he has a high blood sugar before meals, he takes 1 unit of Humalog for every 36 points (2 mmol) above 100 before meals (Chapter 12).

Fig. 6.2

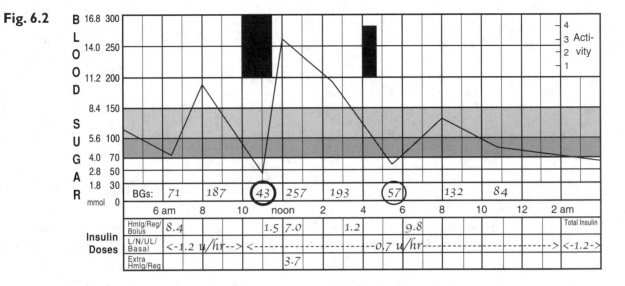

	Breakfast			Lunch			Dinner	
Time	Food	Carb Grams	Time	Food	Carb Grams	Time	Food	Carb Grams
7:00	Cheerios--56 gr.	40	1:00	1 c nonfat milk	13	6:00	pasta and clams	64
	1 c nonfat milk	13		tuna sandwich	34		green salad	11
	strawberries	10		apple--154 grams	23		Chardonnay	6
	2 rye toast	30			70		vanilla ice cream	17
	applebutter	8						98
	poached egg	0						
	AM Snacks	101		Afternoon Snacks			Evening Snacks	
11:00	2 blueberry muffins	70	3:00	crackers	12			
	banana	25		cheese	4			
	diet soda	0	5:00	2 glucose tabs	10			
		95			26			

Day: Saturday   Comments: Biked 21 miles in a.m., but ate too much! Noon, blew my fuse
Date: 9 / 11 / 01   at nursery store clerk ??? 4 pm--helped Fred load dirt into his trailer.

Analysis

On this Saturday, you can see Sam's overall blood sugar control was fairly good. Because the length and intensity of his activity is different from those on a weekday, Sam has been testing his blood sugars more often. Although his readings averaged in the normal range, five of his eight blood sugar tests are out of his desired range.

Sam's early morning basal rate of 1.2 units per hour is higher than during the rest of his day, probably to offset a Dawn Phenomenon (see Chapters 8 and 10). However, this rate appears to be too high since his blood sugar dropped from 129 mg/dl (7.2 mmol) at 3 a.m. (not shown) to 71 mg/dl (3.9 mmol) at 6:30 a.m. at this setting, a 58 point drop over only 3 and 1/2 hours.

Sam took 8.4 units of Humalog 15 minutes before breakfast. Since he uses 1 unit for each 10 grams, this would normally cover 84 grams of carbohydrate. He actually ate 101 grams, probably intending the extra 17 grams to help offset his bike ride later that morning. His mildly elevated blood sugar, 187 mg/dl (10.4 mmol) an hour later, reflects this reduced meal coverage.

On his morning bike ride with the City Cyclers, Sam went 21 miles in an hour and a half at an average speed of 14 miles per hour. From Table 19.1 in Chapter 19, this level of exercise would use a maximum of 70 grams of carbohydrate each hour, or 105 grams for the entire ride.

The extra 17 grams Sam ate at breakfast was not enough to cover the carbs he needed for his bike ride. His low blood sugar at 11 a.m. was a result of too little carbohydrate taken to cover his ride, plus the excess morning basal insulin. Unfortunately, two blueberry muffins and a banana (95 grams of carbs) that he treated the low blood sugar with, plus the stress hormones released by the insulin reaction (his larger circle around the blood sugar of 43 mg/dl (2.4 mmol) indicates this was a major reaction), caused his blood sugar to rise sharply to 257 mg/dl (14.3 mmol). As his appetite subsided and reason returned, he partially corrected the excess carbohydrate for the reaction with a 1.5 unit bolus, enough to cover 15 or so grams.

In his comments, Sam notes that he "blew up" at a store clerk at 11:30 that morning. The clerk may have deserved this response, but it's interesting that the incident occurred as Sam's blood sugar was spiking to the mid-200 range. This sort of irritability can be caused by high blood sugars which decrease oxygen delivery to the frontal cortex, as well as the stress hormone release from his low blood sugar.

At lunch, he took a high blood sugar bolus to lower his still-elevated reading. He wanted to be at 100 mg/dl, so he subtracted 100 from 257 to get his desired drop of 157. Since he drops 36 points per unit, he would normally take an extra 5.2 units in addition to his meal bolus. However, he took only 3.7 extra units to bring the blood sugar down because much of the 1.5 units he'd just taken was still working. This appears to have worked well, as indicated by the drop in his blood sugar to 193 two hours after lunch.

His afternoon snack was covered with a bolus. But helping his neighbor shovel dirt into a trailer was not planned, and Sam didn't take time to eat extra food before starting. He treated the resulting mild low blood sugar at 5:30 p.m. with 15 grams of glucose tablets, enough to raise his blood sugar about 60 points. Dinner appeared to be covered well, producing excellent readings 2 hours after dinner (132) and at bedtime (84).

Suggestions for Sam

1. Retest your nighttime basal rates. Consider reducing the morning basal rate (3 a.m. to 11 a.m.) from 1.2 units/hr to 1.1 and test this new rate at least twice in the next few days to see if the basal is correctly set.

2. When you anticipate any increased activity like cycling or shovelling dirt, use ExCarbs (Chapter 19) to guesstimate how much extra carbohydrate will be needed to cover them. Before the bike ride or a half hour into the ride, he could have eaten a banana along with a cup of milk (approximately 37 grams total), along with drinking or eating another 40 grams or so of carbohydrate during the ride. From Sam's chart, this 77 grams along with the extra 17 grams taken at breakfast probably would have covered the ride. (105 grams = maximum need)

3. Extra blood sugar tests before, during, and after exercise or strenuous work are needed for control.

4. Note any relationship between irritability and blood sugars. If a pattern is recognized, it may avoid some embarrassing personal encounters.

5. Use glucose tablets first for reactions. They raise the blood sugar quickly and by doing so decrease the amount of stress hormones released. They also allow more rational decisions to be made about the quantity and type of food eaten a few minutes later to finish treating the insulin reaction.

6. Eat a bedtime snack when bedtime blood sugars are normal and you have been involved in more activity than usual that day. Extra physical activity can lower the blood sugar for 24 hours or more. Recognizing the extended blood sugar-lowering effect of exercise and that the night basal rate was already too high could have prevented the insulin reaction Sam encountered early Sunday morning (not shown on this chart).

As you fill out your own charts or *Smart Charts*, you may at first have some difficulty in recording all the information. However, by starting with good recording habits, you'll find it much easier to correct any problems you run into later on your pump. With practice, charting becomes a small distraction that pays off by minimizing any reactions and shortening any time spent with high blood sugars.

Be sure to get in the habit of reviewing your charts regularly for patterns, and share them with your physician/health care team. We've analyzed only one chart here due to space constrictions, but you will need to analyze your own over an entire week to find your critical patterns.

Flipping your *Smart Chart* pages back and forth can help you pick up patterns, and looking over your charts regularly will help you evaluate and improve your blood sugar patterns and thereby maximize your health.

"Take notes on the spot, a note is worth a cart-load of recollections."

Ralph Waldo Emerson

Carb Counting

"I never met a carbohydrate I didn't like," is the way many people feel about pasta, potatoes, pastries, fruit, and all the other wonderful foods in this food group. One of the great things about a pump is the opportunity to match any carbohydrate you chance to eat with an exact bolus.

To take advantage of the flexibility a pump affords you, you want a food measuring approach that's as exact and as flexible as your boluses. Counting grams of carbohydrate in foods offers the most precise and flexible approach available today. It's more precise than the exchange system, can be applied directly to the foods in your meal, and is relatively easy to learn and use.

This chapter describes

- Why you want to count carbohydrates
- How carbohydrates affect insulin need
- How to calculate your daily need for carbohydrate
- How to create a healthy meal plan based on carb counting
- Which foods are partially or entirely carbohydrates
- Three ways to count carbohydrate
- The "bigger picture" in healthy eating

The exchange system that many people have learned is based on estimates of the average nutrient values for each of six classes of foods: breads, fruits, vegetables, milk, fats, and meat (or protein). This diet approach is an excellent way to provide balance in nutrient intake, but it is not an exact way to measure carbohydrates. As one pumper put it, "Bagels get bigger every day, but exchanges don't. One half a bagel is still called one bread exchange." If someone who already uses the exchange system has well-controlled blood sugars, this imprecision may not matter, but it may give other people unexpected high blood sugars.

Carb counting is recommended for everyone who needs to improve blood sugar control, and is especially important for people using a pump and needing to adjust carefully to the food they eat.

Why Count Carbs?

Food is made up of three main fuels: carbohydrate, fat, and protein. Carbohydrate is the primary part of food that affects blood sugars. Over 90 percent of the calories from digestible carbohydrates (starches and sugars) end up as glucose. This glucose rapidly raises the blood sugar following a meal. Counting the grams of carbohydrate eaten provides a direct indicator of how high that meal will drive the blood sugar.

To keep the blood sugar at an acceptable level after you eat, the carbs in your food must be balanced with a carb bolus or exercise. Count how many grams of carbohydrate are in the foods you eat and calculate how large a bolus or how much exercise is needed to balance them. Do this by determining how many grams of carb you cover with each unit of insulin or with each half hour of exercise. To determine this ratio, look in Chapter 11.

When the premeal blood sugar is normal, a bolus of Humalog that covers your total carbs is taken 0 to 20 minutes before the meal, or 30 to 45 minutes before eating with Regular. Remember, though, that delaying a meal is one of the most common causes for lows, so do not delay your meal once the bolus is given. Boluses taken to cover carbohydrate generally make up 40 to 50% of the insulin a person takes in 24 hours.

The only time carbs are not covered with a bolus is when carbs are being used to balance exercise or to raise a low blood sugar. For instance, if your blood sugar is 50 mg/dl before a meal, the 10 to 15 grams of carbohydrate that are needed to raise your blood sugar to 100 mg/dl would not be counted when figuring the bolus taken before the meal. Similarly, carbs eaten to replace those burned during a bike ride would not be covered with a bolus.

Counting carbohydrates lets you measure the impact a meal will have on the blood sugar. Though you might not eat them often, even "splurge" foods like ice cream, cake, pie, and candy can be counted and covered by a fast-acting bolus or by exercise so that they don't destroy your hard-won diabetes control.

Although it may not seem this way at first, carb counting is simple and easy to understand. Only one nutrient--carbohydrate--needs to be tracked and measured. Carb counting is especially helpful to those who have a small total daily insulin dose, smaller body size and weight, greater insulin sensitivity, or a higher level of activity.

Carb counting does present some challenges. It involves checking labels or books or perhaps weighing and measuring foods, keeping food records, making various calculations, and testing the blood sugar more often to determine the precise effect the consumed carb has had on the blood sugar. This is especially important when first learning carb counting, and at any time your control is not very good. Attention to so such detail may seem overwhelming to some, but if you keep working at carb counting, it eventually becomes second nature. This is when its real benefits are seen.

Where's The Carbohydrate?

Healthy diets often contain 50 to 60 percent of the day's total calories as carbohydrate. An important exception comes in pregnancy when a 40 percent carbohydrate diet is recommended because blood sugar control is so critical to the health of the child. The American Diabetes Association does not recommend any specific carbohydrate intake, but states that the diet for any person with diabetes needs to be individualized. How much carbohydrate you eat and how you respond to them can only be determined by counting carbs and monitoring how they impact your blood sugar.

Carbohydrate comes from

- Grains (breads, pasta, cereals)
- Fruits and vegetables
- Root crops (potatoes, sweet potatoes, and yams)
- Beer and wine
- Desserts and candies
- Most milk products, except cheese
- -ose foods, like sucrose, fructose, maltose

So What Are Grams?

Carbs are counted as grams. A gram is a unit of weight like pounds or ounces, but because of its small size (it takes 28 grams to make a single ounce), grams can be used to measure components of food accurately. Simply weighing foods does not tell how much carbohydrate they contain.

For example, a cup of milk weighs 224 grams, one rectangular graham cracker (two squares) weighs 14 grams, and a tablespoon of sugar weighs 12 grams. True, but all contain exactly the same amount of carbohydrate: 12 grams. (The milk contains water, the graham crackers contain other non-carbohydrate ingredients, while the sugar is all carbohydrate.) Although their total weights are different, these three food items will require the same bolus to cover them because they each have 12 grams of carbohydrate. Measuring the carb content of foods lets you give exact boluses for the food you eat.

How Many Carbs Do You Need A Day?

Although a healthy diet gets 50 to 60 percent of its calories from complex carbohydrates, most people actually eat only 40 percent of their calories as carbohydrate, with 40 percent as fat and 20 percent as protein. If your current diet has less than the 50 to 60%, you may have difficulty consuming this much carbohydrate at first.

To see whether eating more carbohydrate will be difficult, eat your usual meals for a few days and keep a record of how much carbohydrate you actually take in. Some computer software programs will conveniently analyze your daily diet for you. If you are eating significantly less carbohydrate than that recommended in Workspace 7.1, try increasing your carbohydrate intake by 10 percent while reducing fat and protein calories by the same amount. Because carbohydrate plays such a major role in setting your insulin doses, it is best to gradually change how much carbohydrate you eat. You may find that abruptly increasing the amount of carbohydrate you eat makes blood sugar control more difficult.

A higher carb intake helps reduce fat and protein calories in the diet. Less fat and protein in your diet lessens your risks for heart disease and kidney disease respectively, risks which are quite high in people with diabetes. Over 70 percent of people with Type 2 diabetes, for instance, die as a result of cardiovascular disease, while some 30 percent of those with Type 1 diabetes die directly or indirectly from kidney disease. If you find you have a problem balancing your carbs with boluses, be sure to discuss how to match boluses to carbs with your physician or dietician.

Your daily carbohydrate goal is based on how many total calories you need. A person who needs 2000 calories a day would get 1000 to 1200 of those calories from the carbohydrate in breads, grains, vegetables, fruits, low-fat milk, and so on. Since there are four calories in each gram of carbohydrate, a person eating 2000 calories per day would need between 250 to 300 grams (1000 calories divided by four to 1200 calories divided by four) of carbohydrate.

That number becomes the basis of a carb counting meal plan. The total amount of carbohydrate for the day is divided among the meals and snacks a person normally eats. The box on page 65 shows three examples of how 225 grams of total daily carbohydrate can be divided among meals and snacks. Your own pattern can be based on your personal preferences and needs.

One nice thing about an insulin pump is that snacks are no longer required. Once the background insulin has been correctly set, you have the freedom to enjoy snacks and cover them with a bolus when you want, not when your insulin says you must. Use Workspace 7.2 to divide your carbs into daily meals and snacks.

Healthy Carbohydrates

In a healthy diet, most carbohydrate comes from nutrient-dense foods like whole grains, fruits, legumes, vegetables, nonfat or low fat milk, and yogurt. Nutrient-dense foods have a high volume of nutrients like vitamins, minerals, fiber, and protein in proportion to their calorie content. They also tend to be lower on the glycemic index. Low nutrient foods such as candy and regular sodas contain carbohydrate, but they lack the other nutrients your cells require to remain healthy. Furthermore, since they

Workspace 7.1 How Many Carbs Do You Need A Day?

Fill in the blanks below to determine how many grams of carbohydrate you need a day.

1. First determine your desired weight in pounds from Table 7.1, or if overweight, a 10% reduction is ideal.

    My desired weight is _____ lbs.

2. Choose a calorie factor that best describes your activity level from Table 7.2.

    My calorie factor from Table 7.2 equals _____

3. Next determine your total daily calorie need:

    _____ lbs. multiplied by _____ equals _____ calories
    my desired weight   my calorie factor   # of calories needed a day

4. Then divide your total daily calories by 8* to determine the total grams of carbohydrate you need each day with 50 percent of calories as carbohydrate:

    _____ calories ÷ 8 equals _____ grams
    calories/day   grams of carbs/day

    * 1/2 of calories as carbohydrate and 1/4 gram per calorie
    Consult with your dietician for specific help.

Table 7.1 Optimum Weights For Men And Women (Any Age):

Height	Weight in pounds
4' 10"	91–119
4' 11"	94–124
5' 0"	97–128
5' 1"	101–132
5' 2"	104–137
5' 3"	107–141
5' 4"	111–146
5' 5"	114–150
5' 6"	118–155
5" 7"	121–160
5' 8"	125–164
5' 9'	129–169
5" 10"	132–174
5" 11"	136–179
6' 0"	140–184

Table 7.2 Calorie Factors For Different Levels Of Activity

Activity Level	Calorie Factor Male	Calorie Factor Female
Very Sedentary: Limited activity, slow walking, mostly sitting.	13	11.5
Sedentary: Recreational activities include walking, bowling, fishing, or similar activities.	14	12.5
Moderately Active: Recreational activities include 18 hole golf, aerobic dancing, pleasure swimming, etc.	15	13.5
Active: Greater than 20 minutes of jogging, swimming, competitive tennis or similar activities more than three times per week.	16	14.5
Super Active: At least one hour of vigorous activity such as football, weight training, or full-court basketball four or more days per week.	17	15.5

What About Fat?

Food contains three different fuels--carbohydrate, fat, and protein--and all contribute glucose to the blood, but the contributions are not equal. The fat in certain foods, for instance, may delay absorption of carbohydrate from the intestine and reduce the expected rise in blood sugars.[48] The fat in old-fashioned ice cream, which has a low glycemic index (raises the blood sugar slowly), is a good example of this. On the other hand, certain high fat meals create a rapid, temporary state of insulin resistance for up to 8 to 16 hours, making blood sugars rise late.[49,50] Many meat pizzas will create this unexpected rise long after they were eaten and the bolus is gone.

High fat diets lead to weight gain and the permanent insulin resistance that is common in Type 2 diabetes, particularly in those prone to an apple figure or male pattern obesity.[51,52,53] Insulin resistance makes it harder for sugar to be used as fuel. At the same time, the high fat diet causes extra fat and glucose to be produced and released into the bloodstream. People who have Type 1 diabetes due to insulin deficiency can develop the apple shape and insulin resistance characteristic of Type 2 diabetes as they age. Although the effect of fat on blood sugars after most high fat meals or snacks is small,[54] dietary fat, especially saturated and hydrogenated or trans fat, should be reduced for better health.

What About Protein?

Normal portions of dietary protein have little impact on sugars.[55] Making up only 10 to 20 percent of calories in most diets, protein determines less than a tenth of the total blood sugar control.

Larger quantities of protein, however, can cause blood sugars to rise. Some 50 percent of protein calories are slowly converted to glucose over a period of several hours, so an eight-ounce steak or several ounces of cheese may cause blood sugars to rise 4 to 12 hours later. Following a high-protein dinner, for instance, blood sugars may not peak until the following morning.

To cover this delayed effect from high protein meals, a small increase in the evening and night basals might be considered but only if such a meal has consistently raised the next morning's blood sugar in the past. Breaking the meal bolus into two smaller boluses, the second one taken two or three hours after the meal, may also work to control the blood sugar. A better plan for blood sugar control (and better protection for the kidneys) is to limit how often this much protein is eaten. Talk to your doctor and dietician if you think your intake of protein is more than normal and might be affecting your blood sugar.

often contain simple sugar and refined grains, they have a high glycemic index and are more likely to cause the blood sugar to spike.

Nutrient-dense foods like brown rice and broccoli are better for

Three Ways To Divide Carbs Through The Day

Example 1:   Big breakfast & lunch, light dinner & bedtime snack
Example 2:   Light breakfast and frequent snacks
Example 3:   Carbs evenly divided among meals

Meal or Snack	Example 1	Example 2	Example 3
Breakfast	75 grams	30 grams	75 grams
Morning snack		15 grams	
Lunch	70 grams	45 grams	75 grams
Afternoon snack		30 grams	
Dinner	40 grams	75 grams	75 grams
Bedtime snack	40 grams	30 grams	

This example is based on a total daily carb need of **225 grams**

your health as well as better for your blood sugars. Eating nutrient dense carbs is important for your health, but always remember that it is the total amount of carbohydrate in a meal that determines what impact a meal will have on your blood sugar.

How To Count Carbohydrates

A few foods like table sugar and lollipops are entirely carbohydrate. Their weight on a gram scale is exactly the same as the number of grams of carbohydrate they contain. Most foods, however, have only part of their total weight as carbohydrate. The carb content of these foods can be determined by food labels,

Workspace 7.2 Carbs For Meals & Snacks

Once you know how many carbs you need a day from Workspace 7.1, decide how you want to split up your total carbohydrates for the day into different meals:

breakfast _____ grams

AM snack _____ grams

lunch _____ grams

PM snack _____ grams

dinner _____ grams

eve. snack _____ grams

reference books, or a scale and a list of carb factors.

Like any new skill, counting grams of carbohydrate will take a couple of weeks to master. You'll need to consult books and weigh and measure foods consistently. As time passes, you'll train your eye to estimate accurately both serving sizes and weights, whether eating out or at home. As you look up the foods you commonly eat, make a list of them for easy reference.

Eventually, you'll be able to look at a piece of fruit, a bowl of pasta, or a plate of stir-fried veggies and rice at home or in your favorite restaurant and accurately estimate its carbohydrate count, without weighing, measuring or looking up a thing. This, of course, is easier if you tend to eat the same thing often, as many people do. Be patient but persistent as you develop this skill. When you can adjust your boluses precisely to the carbohydrates you eat, it will be worth all the effort.

Carb Counting And The 500 Rule

Table 11.1 in Chapter 11 can be used to determine how many carbs are covered by each unit of Humalog or Regular based on your total daily insulin dose or TDD. The 500 Rule, determined from clinical experience, says that the number of grams of carbohydrate covered by one unit of Humalog equals 500 divided by the TDD (total daily insulin dose).

For example, someone using 50 total units of insulin a day will need a unit of Humalog for every ten grams of carbohydrate (500 divided by 50 = 10). If they eat three slices of bread and each has 15 grams of carbohydrate, they would use a bolus of 4.5 units to cover this 45 grams. This assumes, of course, that the basal rates are already correctly set.

Equipment

Carb counting requires some measuring equipment, such as a digital gram scale and measuring cups and spoons. Scales measure weight, while measuring cups and spoons measure volume. For some foods there is a big difference. For example, ten ounces of Cheerios® by volume (1 1/4 cups) is equal to one ounce by weight (28 grams). Many nutrition labels and food composition tables give both types of measure, but some give only one.

Measuring Cups and Spoons: Accurate measuring cups and spoons are available in many different places and price ranges. Use a glass measuring container that allows you to "sight" across the top for measuring liquids and a different one that lets you scrape a knife across the top to get the exact measure for dry items such as cereal and rice.

Gram scales: A gram scale measures the actual weight of a food in grams. A good scale will weigh food accurately within one or two grams. Look also for a tare feature that allows you to zero out the weight of containers. This lets you pour your food directly into the serving bowl, and eliminates the hassle of weighing foods on the scale and then moving them into your bowl.

If you can afford a few extra dollars, a computerized gram scale can save a lot of effort. These scales are pre-programmed with the percentage of nutrients contained in each food. You simply enter a code into the scale for a food from a list of codes, and then place that food on the scale. The scale can then give you the total weight of the food, and the grams of carbohydrate, fat, protein, cholesterol and calories it contains.

Several brands of scales are available, ranging in price from $50 to $80 for simple digital scales to $130 for a scale containing an internal database of foods that can also be programmed with your own foods. Scales can be found in gourmet and kitchen shops, or online discount retailers like the Diabetes Mall.

Carbs in foods can be determined in three ways: food labels, nutrition books and cookbooks, or gram scales.

Food Labels

All packaged foods today have a "Nutrition Facts" label on them. This label contains information about the nutritional quantities in that product, including the number of calories and the grams of carbohydrate, protein, and fat contained in one serving. These labels are great for carb counting because they give the exact number of grams of carbohydrate contained in a serving. An example is given below.

If you're eating a food that has all the information you need on the label, you can calculate insulin coverage easily. For example, an 8-ounce carton of Elsie's Lowfat Yogurt has a label that tells you that an 8-ounce serving has 17 grams of carbohydrate. Once you know this and also know how many grams of carbohydrate are covered by one unit of insulin for you from Chapter 11, you can figure out the bolus you need to cover this food. If the serving you eat varies from the serving size listed on the package, you will have to weigh or measure your actual serving and do some calculations.

On labels, focus on the Total Carb usually in bold, but also pay attention to fiber. Although fiber is carbohydrate, it has little effect on your blood sugar. If a food has 4 or more grams of fiber in a portion, subtract the grams of fiber from the Total Carb grams before calculating your bolus.

Elsie's Lowfat Yogurt		
Nutrition Facts		
Serving Size 1 cup (225 g)		
Servings Per Container 4		
Amount Per Serving		
Calories 120	Fat Cal 0	
		% Daily Value
Total Fat 0g		0%
Saturated Fat 0g		0%
Cholesterol 5 mg		2%
Sodium 180 mg		8%
Total Carbohydrate 17g		6%
Dietary Fiber 0g		0%
Sugars 17g		
Protein 12g		

Advantage: Very easy.

What you need: Food labels, occasionally a measuring cup, and a calculator for calculating the carbs in the amount you plan to eat, especially if it differs from the portion size given on the label.

What To Do: Food labels contain all the information needed to do carb counting. Just be sure your serving is the same size as the serving on the label, or do some calculating.

Nutrition Books and Cookbooks

Nutrition books and brochures, just like nutrition labels, describe the amount of carbohydrate in a typical serving size of each food. If what you eat varies from this serving size, you will need to weigh or measure your actual serving, and then do the necessary calculations to learn how many grams of carbohydrate are in your own serving. Cookbooks often have the number of grams of carbohydrate in a portion size. Again you may have to calculate the number of carbs in your serving if it is not the same as the portion size.

Advantage: Nutrition books can provide information useful for eating out and are an easy way to look up many brand name foods. Cookbooks are great for counting carbohydrates when preparing meals at home.

What you need: Books and occasionally measuring cups, spoons, and scales to determine serving size.

Example: Two servings of Wild Rice	**Uncle Bob's Wild Rice**

Example: Two servings of Wild Rice

1. Look at the label. Let's say you want to eat a cup of Uncle Bob's Wild Rice, but a serving size is a half cup.

2. Look on the label for the number of carbohydrates in one serving (a half cup).

3. Multiply this number (27 grams) by two to determine the carbohydrate you will be eating:

Carbs in a half cup portion = 27 grams

Times 2 for one cup serving = X 2

Total Carbs = 54 grams

Uncle Bob's Wild Rice

Nutrition Facts
Serving Size 1/2 cup cooked (38 g)
Servings Per Container 8

Amount Per Serving
Calories 130   Fat Cal 0

% Daily Value

Total Fat 0g	0%
Saturated Fat 0g	0%
Cholesterol 0 mg	0%
Sodium 0 mg	0%
Total Carb 27g	6%
Dietary Fiber 0g	0%
Sugars 3g	
Protein 4g	

What To Do: Look for books and cookbooks in the "Nutrition and Diet" section of your local bookstore, library, or online sources like the Diabetes Mall (www.diabetesnet.com). Look also for recipes with carbohydrate content in the "Food" section of your local newspaper.

A Gram Scale or Computer Scale

Most carbohydrate foods contain only a percentage of their total weight as carbohydrate. When you eat a food like fruit that has no label, you have to calculate the grams of carbohydrate in your serving. You can do this by weighing the food on a gram scale and then multiplying its total weight by a "carb factor," which is the percentage of total weight that is carbohydrate.

If you weigh food on a computer scale, just put in the code for the food, push the button for "carbohydrate" and the computer scale does the calculation for you. You can even program computerized scales to give you the percentage of carbohydrate of your favorite combination foods such as stir-fried vegetables with rice.

Advantage: Convenient for measuring carbs in odd-sized foods like fruits, unsliced bread, cereals, or casseroles.

What you need: A gram scale, a calculator, and a list of carb factors like those in Appendix A at the back of this book, or a computer scale.

What To Do: To find the amount of carbohydrate in a portion of food

Gram Scale:

1. Weigh the food to find its total weight in grams.
2. Find the food's carb factor in one of the food groups listed in Appendix A.
3. Multiply the food's total weight in grams by its carb factor.
4. This number is the number of grams of carbohydrate you are eating.

Example: Measure the carbs in cooked spaghetti.

With a standard gram scale: Use a gram scale and a list of carb factors to determine carbs:

1. Zero out your plate on the scale and place the amount of cooked spaghetti you want to eat on it.

2. Let's say the portion you want has a total weight of 200 grams on the scale. From Appendix A, you find that cooked plain spaghetti has a carb factor of 0.26, meaning 26 percent of its weight is carbohydrate.

3. Now multiply the spaghetti's total weight by its carb factor.

Weight of spaghetti	=	200 grams
Carb factor for spaghetti	=	X 0.26
Total carbs in your portion	=	52 grams of carbohydrate

4. So, when you eat 200 grams of cooked spaghetti, you'll actually eat 52 grams of carbohydrate.

With a computer gram scale: Computerized gram scales already contain information about the nutrition content of spaghetti and other foods:

1. Zero out your plate on the scale.

2. Enter the food code for spaghetti into the scale.

3. Put the portion of spaghetti you want onto your plate.

4. Press the carbohydrate key on the scale.

5. Read the grams of carbohydrate in the spaghetti.

Is Carb Counting The Only Way?

No. There are other ways to improve your control with food. Other ways to measure the impact a meal will have on your blood sugar include the exchange system, counting calories, and the TAG (total available glucose) system.

Food exchange lists give the approximate carbohydrate content of foods. In some cases, the exchange system will describe your particular food accurately, and in some cases, it doesn't. Here are examples that illustrate this inconsistency. The exchange value of one slice of bread is 15 grams of carb.

Example 1: A slice of Wonder bread (1 bread exchange) = 15 grams of carb

Actual carb value   =   15 grams of carb

Here the values are the same, so there's no problem.

Example 2:   A slice of Lieken bread (1 bread exchange) = 29 grams of carb

In the second example the actual carb value of Lieken bread, which is similar in size but denser than Wonder bread, is nearly twice the exchange value. With most food items, the differences between the exchange system value and the actual grams of carbohydrate won't be this large, but when estimating your carb bolus, if the carbohydrate content of several items in a meal is estimated using exchanges, the differences that may occur can total a miscalculation large enough to cause control problems.

The exchange system divides foods into broad categories like breads, meats, and fruits, and then gives portion sizes having about the same nutritional value. If the exchange system, counting calories, or even your own intuition is working well for you, don't change a thing. On the other hand, if your control is not what you desire, or you're interested in a more flexible, logical, and exact approach to blood sugar control, learn carb counting.

Weight Gain

Horror stories about people gaining weight when they begin to control their blood sugars certainly exist. However, weight gain does not have to happen with improved control. The road to real blood sugar control lies in eating what you need, and adjusting your insulin to handle that amount of food. You don't want to give up good diabetes control just because of a weight gain, but also realize you can lose excess weight while maintaining good control if you follow a healthy, sensible diet at every meal and stay active.

With your sugar in good control, your body behaves just like it did before you had diabetes. If you eat too much, you gain weight. If you eat less, you lose weight.

Keep track of your weight and your appetite. These tell you whether you're actually eating the right amount of food. Keep the fat and protein calories at moderate levels. Research has shown that meals that are higher in fat actually are less satisfying and will trigger hunger sooner than high carb meals, especially complex carbs. Maybe you just don't need all the food that you're consuming. Focus on an appropriate carbohydrate and calorie intake!

The Bigger Nutrition Picture

When you have mastered the art of carbohydrate counting, and can figure your insulin-to-carb ratio, you will be an expert in balancing your insulin and food intake to achieve blood sugar control. As important as that is, however, blood sugar control is not the only health goal you have. Your overall health depends on eating a wide variety of nutrient-rich foods.

The amount and type of fat in your diet appears to be very important to health. High intake of saturated fats and trans or hydrogenated fats has been associated with greater risks for heart disease, cancer, and obesity. Heart disease is especially common in people with diabetes, where a two- to six-fold increase is seen. A fat intake of no more than 20 percent to 30 percent of total calories is recommended by the American Heart Association and the American Dietetic Association. This focus on reducing fat intake, especially saturated and hydrogenated fats, may be one reason for the gradual reduction in the number of heart attacks over the last few years.

Most people cut back by cutting down on fats added to foods (butter, margarine, sour cream, salad dressings, oils and shortening used for frying, etc.). They also choose protein foods that are lower in fat or that contain better types of fat (fish, skinless chicken, nonfat milk, and nonfat cheese products, for example). Diets that are lower in animal protein also have been shown to slow the development and progression of diabetic kidney disease. Because about 30 to 35 percent of people with Type 1 diabetes develop kidney disease, keeping red meat portions smaller is highly recommended, and this automatically lowers fat intake.

After talking about reducing our consumption of greasy favorites, let's talk about a change in the diabetes diet that is good news. As most of us remember, the dietary harangue in the past was "No Sugar!" This taboo has been relaxed in recent years as blood sugar testing has shown that it's possible to retain glycemic control when eating some "splurge foods" if we know how to manage their sometimes hefty carbohydrate content. This has become easier since the introduction of faster insulins.

Sugar is no longer banned from coffee, nor jelly from toast, nor an occasional small piece of pie from the dinner table. It appears that it may, in fact, be healthier to have a small amount of applebutter (which has some sugar but no fat in it) on your waffle rather than the butter or margarine used in the past.

No one with or without diabetes really benefits nutritionally from an excess of high-calorie, low-nutrient foods. However, small amounts of sweets can add flavor to a diet and, if chosen wisely, make avoiding fatty foods easier. Be careful though: sugar almost always travels with fat. For instance, a chocolate candy bar gets about 60 percent of its calories from fat!

If you find that sweets are addictive for you and a little is never enough, you may find it easier to eliminate splurge foods entirely. Whether you include some sweets in your meals or not, the key to blood sugar control is to determine the amount of carbohydrate in your food and cover it with an appropriate amount of insulin. This and a nutrient-rich, low-fat, low-protein diet, is a vital part of any healthy lifestyle.

Two elderly women are at a Catskill Mountain Resort and one of them says, "Boy, the food at this place is really terrible." The other one says, "Yeah, I know, and such small portions."

Woody Allen

The Glycemic Index

The glycemic index is a well-researched ranking of carbohydrate foods based on how quickly they are digested and how quickly and how high they raise the blood sugar.[90-93] Knowing this can be very helpful for preventing unwanted spikes after meals and raising low blood sugars quickly.

For example, when your blood sugar is already low or rapidly dropping due to exercise, you want carbs that will raise it quickly. On the other hand, to prevent a gradual blood sugar drop during a few hours of mild activity, you might prefer to eat carbs with a low glycemic index and long action time. If your blood sugar tends to spike after breakfast, you may want to change your cereal to one with a lower glycemic index. Lower glycemic index foods also help to prevent overnight drops in the blood sugar because their action lasts for a longer period of time.

A food's glycemic index is a number that indicates the food's effect on the blood sugar. The number shows how quickly that food will raise the blood sugar relative to the action of glucose, which is the fastest carbohydrate. Glucose is given a value of 100, and then other carbs are given a number relative to glucose. Fast carbs have higher numbers and are great for raising low blood sugars or for covering brief periods of intense exercise. Slower carbs have lower numbers and are the best choices to maintain good control in your day-to-day diet.

Table 7.3 provides glycemic index values for a wide variety of foods. If you prefer to use white bread as your standard instead of glucose, simply multiply the glycemic index numbers in the table by 1.42. For instance, glucose would have a glycemic index of 142 on a white-bread-based glycemic index.

A food's ranking is compiled from more than one research study if possible. More than one glycemic index list exists. Each list will be close to, but may not be identical to other lists. The actual impact a food has on your blood sugar also will depend on factors other than the glycemic index, like ripeness, cooking time, fiber and fat content, time of day eaten, blood insulin level, and recent activity. Use the glycemic index as just one of the many tools you have available to improve your control.

Research studies have drawn mixed conclusions on how well the glycemic index measures a food's effect on blood sugar control. However, many pumpers have found they can improve their blood sugar control through wise use of this information. If you are using a continuous blood glucose monitor, you can create your own personalized glycemic index based on how different foods affect your blood sugar.

An excellent book that provides more information on this topic is **The Glucose Revolution**. The authors of this highly readable and scientifically sound book are respected nutrition experts who have taken their findings from 15-20 years of research regarding hundreds of people's blood sugar response to foods.

The waist is a terrible thing to mind.
Ziggy (Tom Wilson)

Table 7.3 The Glycemic Index

Foods are compared to glucose, which ranks 100. Higher numbers indicate faster absorption and a faster rise in the blood sugar, while lower numbers indicate a slower rise.

Breads		Cereals		Drinks		Pasta	
baguette, Frnch	95	All Bran™	51	apple juice	40	fettuccini	32
hamburger bun	61	Bran Buds +psyll	45	colas	65	linguini	50
muffins		Bran Flakes™	74	Gatorade™	78	macaroni	46
blueberry	59	Cheerios™	74	grapefruit juice	48	spagh, 5 m boil	33
oat & raisin	54	Corn Chex™	83	orange juice	46	spagh, 15m boil	44
pita	57	Cornflakes™	83	pineapple juice	46	spagh, prot enr	28
pizza, cheese	60	Frosted Flakes™	55	**Fruit**		vermicelli	35
pumpernickel	49	Grapenuts™	67	apple	38	**Root Crops**	
sourdough	54	muesli, natural	54	apricots	57	French fries	75
rye	64	oatmeal, old fash	48	banana	56	pot, new, boiled	59
white	70	Puffed Wheat™	67	cantalope	65	pot, red, baked	93
wheat	68	Raisin Bran™	73	cherries	22	pot, sweet	52
Beans		Rice Krispies™	82	grapefruit	25	pot, wht, boiled	63
baked	44	Shredded Wht™	67	grapes	46	pot, wht, mash	70
butter, boiled	33	Special K™	54	orange	43	yam	54
garbanzo, boiled	34	**Milk Products**		peach	42	**Snacks**	
kidney, boiled	29	chocolate milk	35	pear	58	chocolate bar	49
kidney, canned	52	ice cream, van	60	pineapple	66	corn chips	72
lima, boiled	32	ice milk, van	50	plums	39	croissant	67
pinto, boiled	39	milk	30	raisins	64	doughnut	76
red lentils, boil	27	soy	31	**Soups/Vegetables**		jelly beans	80
soy, boiled	16	yogurt, fruit	36	corn, sweet	56	Life Savers™	70
Crackers		yogurt, plain	14	green pea soup	66	oatmeal cookie	57
graham	74	**Sugars**		green pea, frzn	47	potato chips	56
rice cakes	80	fructose	22	lentil soup	44	Power Bars™	58
rye	68	honey	62	tomato soup	38	pretzels	83
soda	72	maltose	105			vanilla wafers	77
Wheat Thins™	67	table sugar	64				

Basals And Boluses

To recap briefly, in past chapters you have learned:

- How pump therapy works
- Why normal blood sugars are so important
- How to use charts to find your blood sugar patterns
- How to count carbohydrates

This basic foundation has given you the tools to begin taking control of your blood sugars.

In this chapter you will learn:

- Insulin's roles in control
- The difference between basal and bolus insulin usage
- How to use basal rates to provide the background insulin needed
- How to use boluses to cover carbohydrates
- How to use boluses to bring down high blood sugars

Insulin Delivery

Because insulin has many roles, a critical level of insulin must always be available in the bloodstream and at the cell-. In the normal pancreas, beta cells deliver the exact amounts of insulin needed to help glucose move from the blood into fat, muscle, and liver cells without depleting the blood of its glucose supply. Enough glucose must be left in the blood so that the brain and nervous system can receive the fuel they need for their vital functions.

To balance insulin's actions, the body depends on the release of other hormones, like epinephrine, growth hormone, and cortisol. These other so-called counter-regulatory hormones balance insulin by releasing glucose from glycogen stores within liver and muscle cells to prevent blood sugars from going too low.

When functioning normally, the pancreas releases insulin in two ways to cover two distinct needs:

- as a constant background release to maintain ongoing metabolism, and

- as short spurts or boluses that cover carbohydrate intake in meals or snacks.

Of course, other things may change how much insulin is needed, like an infection (more insulin) or exercise (less insulin), but understanding the two needs above is critical for understanding how to use insulin to control blood sugars.

Figure 8.1 shows a normal release of insulin into the blood over 24 hours. The darker band at the bottom of the figure represents a relatively constant release of background or basal insulin. Background delivery adjusts naturally, of course, for exercise, the Dawn phenomenon, stress, and other factors.

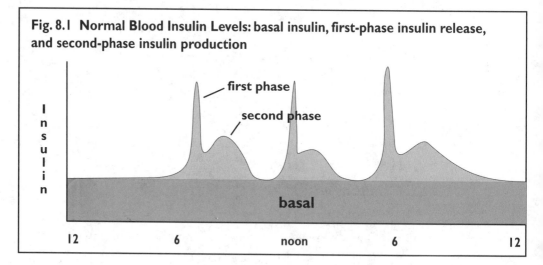

Fig. 8.1 Normal Blood Insulin Levels: basal insulin, first-phase insulin release, and second-phase insulin production

As soon as food is eaten, a quick release of "first phase" insulin can be seen. In the figure, this quick release is shown as happening three times a day, but if you eat more often, it happens more often. This fast insulin release in the first 15 minutes after eating comes from insulin already stored within the beta cells of the pancreas. This quick release is then followed by a more gradual second phase over the next hour and a half to three hours as insulin production rises within the beta cells.

In contrast to normal insulin delivery by a healthy pancreas, a pump has a basal release for ongoing metabolism, carb boluses to cover carb intake, and high blood sugar boluses to lower high readings when basals or carb boluses have been inadequate. The basal rate can be modified for various needs. Carb and high blood sugar boluses are actually delivered as rounded half-ellipses, rather than as the first and second phase spikes seen in Fig. 8.1. A pump has no equivalent first-phase insulin release, although the speed of Humalog insulin helps to approximate it.

One of the great advantages of an insulin pump is its ability to cover the three needs separately. This allows independent, accurate testing of each part of the control process.

Testing the basal rates and boluses usually can be completed within the first month of pump use. Once correctly set, basals and boluses may occasionally need retesting to accommodate changes in weight or activity or when blood sugar control is less than desired. This retesting usually can be completed within a few days to regain control.

How To Find Your Insulin Doses

The goal in pump therapy is to keep your blood sugars as normal as possible. Reaching this goal requires that you test and set your insulin doses in five steps that are described below, with testing procedures outlined in Chapters 10, 11, and 12. Whenever possible, follow these steps in the sequence given. You may want to review the PumpFormance Checklist in Chapter 2, or read the entire book for a better understanding of what you will be doing, and then return to Chapter 10 where testing actually begins. Here is how it works:

First: Determine your **Total Daily Dose** of insulin or **TDD**. Once you know your average TDD, you can quickly estimate your starting basal rates and boluses with Table 10.1 in Chapter 10. How to quickly adjust your TDD when control is less than desired, or for longer periods of exercise, or for a premenstrual rise in blood sugars, is also outlined.

Second: Test your **basal rates**. Basal rates are always tested before boluses because a correct basal allows you to keep your blood sugars normal when you are sleeping and when you skip or delay meals. You must establish these background rates before you can accurately set boluses. Testing night and day basals is covered in Chapter 10.

Third: Test your **carb boluses**. Before testing, you need to know how to count the grams of carbohydrate in your meals, covered in Chapter 7. Setting and testing your carb coverage is covered in Chapter 11. First, you'll decide what your insulin-to-carb ratio is, or exactly how much carbohydrate is covered by each unit of insulin. Then you'll test it to see if the ratio is accurate. Once your basal rates are set correctly, balancing carbohydrates in your meals with precise boluses allows you to eat meals without losing control of your blood sugars.

Fourth: Test your **high blood sugar boluses**. When you have a high blood sugar, you want to bring it down quickly so you can safely return to normal. How to test this is outlined in Chapter 12. First, you determine how many points your blood sugar drops on each unit of Humalog, and then you can set up your own personalized table for correcting high blood sugars with supplemental boluses. The table can be used as needed to lower high blood sugars to a normal reading.

Fifth: Learn how to use the **unused bolus rule** when boluses overlap. Described in Chapter 13, this rule helps you estimate how much insulin is still working from recent boluses. Knowing this allows you to avoid giving too much insulin in situations where boluses overlap.

For people who exercise regularly, the information for exercise in Chapters 18 and 19 can help in adjusting basals and boluses appropriately. Learn to use ExCarbs to balance exercise. Because exercise affects your blood sugar, extra carbohydrate, less insulin, or both are needed when you're engaged in increased physical activity.

These five steps provide the major tools needed to set your basal rate and boluses for great blood sugar control on your pump. Let's look more closely at what your basal rates and boluses do before we begin to test them.

Beware Of Lows Following Pump Startup

When first starting on a pump, both you and your doctor may be surprised by how quickly your total daily insulin dose (TDD) drops. As your blood sugars improve from better insulin delivery on your pump, your insulin doses may need to be reduced within the first one to four days of use to prevent low blood sugars.

On a pump, you have a new ability to maintain normal blood sugars, but don't overdo it. Your goal is to stay between 70 to 120 mg/dl (3.9 to 6.7 mmol) before meals and no higher than 140 to 180 mg/dl (7.8 to 10 mmol) after meals. Be willing to set realistic goals, to pace yourself, and to celebrate small steps as you move toward a normal range.

Most importantly, check your blood sugar at least 7 times a day and anytime you suspect it may be going low. If you have access to a continuous monitoring device, use it. As your physician/health care team gives you more responsibility in adjusting your basals and boluses, make these adjustments only after adequate testing. Adjust your insulin doses gradually and in agreement with your physician/health care team's recommendations.

What Is Basal Insulin?

Insulin's roles in the body include helping glucose enter certain cells, helping to regulate the production and release of fats as fuel, and helping some of the amino acids that create enzymes and structural proteins to enter cells. Cells need a background or basal insulin supply at all times to accomplish these tasks. Of your total daily insulin dose, you need about half as basal insulin.[56]

The basal insulin delivery from a pump provides this background insulin around the clock. People often require minor adjustments in their basal rates during the day to balance the changing output of counter-regulatory or stress hormones. For example, most people require a small upward basal adjustment during the early morning hours to counteract extra growth hormone production during the next few morning hours, called the Dawn Phenomenon. If extra insulin is not provided at this time, the blood sugar rises.

For simplicity, many people start with a single basal rate as they begin insulin pump therapy. This single rate can then be tested to see if it needs to be adjusted. Research shows that some 70% of people have a Dawn Phenomenon, and for this reason basal rates that vary slightly through the day and night often work better than one rate. A bicyclic pattern is usually an effective basal pattern for this, with lower rates during the middle of the night and the afternoon, and higher rates during the early morning and dinner hours.

Basal insulin delivery from a pump is superior to injections in controlling the Dawn Phenomenon. This is true for controlling waking blood sugars[57] and also for blood sugars in the early afternoon hours.[58] On average, a 20% increase in the early morning basal rate is needed to offset a Dawn Phenomenon.[59] The increased basal need for a Dawn Phenomenon often requires only an additional 0.1 or 0.2 unit/hour (u/hr), such as a rise from 0.6 u/hr in the middle of the night to 0.7 u/hr or 0.8 u/hr during the hours of 2 a.m. to 9 a.m. A large increase in basal rates is rarely needed if a smaller increase is begun early, usually at 1 or 2 a.m. using Humalog insulin.

> **Control Tip: First Things First**
>
> For great control, focus first on setting up your nighttime basal rates so that your overnight blood sugar is flat and you wake up with a normal blood sugar in the morning. Next test and adjust the daytime basal rates, then carb coverage, and finally your point drop for safely lowering highs.

When the basal rate has been correctly set, the blood sugar remains level or drops slightly during fasting. A good target for most pumpers is to have the blood sugar drop no more than 0 to 30 mg/dl during eight hours of sleep, and no more than 0 to 30 mg/dl during any five hour period of the waking hours.

It is important to realize that basal rates are very different from boluses in how they impact your blood sugar. Compared to the quick effect of changing a bolus, a change in the basal rate has little effect. For instance, a bolus of Humalog will begin to lower blood sugars in about 20 minutes. But a basal rate increase is much smaller and usually has almost no impact on the blood sugars until 90 to 120 minutes have passed.[60] This is why stopping the basal insulin delivery is never recommended when treating a low blood sugar; it simply takes too long to have an impact.

Remember to set and test your basal rates before estimating your bolus insulin doses. For instance, if a basal rate is too high and a meal and meal bolus are skipped, low blood sugar symptoms begin shortly afterward. An accurate meal bolus also would be smaller than expected.

With the basal rate set too low, just the opposite happens. A person would require larger than normal boluses for meals, and when meals are skipped, the blood sugar would climb as the hours pass. Basal rates must be set correctly before you can determine carb or high blood sugar boluses.

What Are Boluses?

Once your basal rates are set correctly to cover background need, short bursts of insulin called boluses can be used to cover the other two needs:

- carb boluses to cover the carbohydrate in snacks and meals
- high blood sugar boluses to lower high blood sugars

Carb Boluses

The amount of carbohydrate that will be eaten in a meal determines how much bolus insulin is needed to cover it. The more carbohydrate, the larger the bolus needed to balance it.

Because pumps do not yet deliver insulin directly into the blood, it is important to correctly time carb boluses. Humalog, for instance, begins working in 10 to 15 minutes, peaks in about an hour and a half, and is gone in about 3.5 hours. Fortunately, this closely matches the digestion time for most meals, which means boluses can be given immediately before eating and still keep blood sugars low after meals. Whenever possible, a 20 minute lead time is better, because it lets the bolused insulin begin to appear in the blood at about the same time as quickly digested carbohydrates. Humalog's effect is gone about the same time the food has been digested.

The action time for Regular insulin is slower and does not match the digestion of food as well as Humalog. Regular starts in 20 minutes, peaks in 3 hours, and keeps working for 6 to 8 hours after a bolus. It is slower to start and continues to lower blood sugars for 2 to 4 hours after most meals are digested. Regular, therefore, needs to be bolused at least 30 minutes before a meal to avoid the spiking in blood sugar often seen 1 to 2 hours after eating. It is also more likely to cause delayed low blood sugars.

Take a carbohydrate bolus every time you eat carbohydrate except:

- when eating carbs to correct a low blood sugar (see Chapter 15),
- when compensating for extra physical activity with carbohydrate (see Chapter 19), or
- when you are unsure if you can keep food down due to nausea or vomiting.

For instance, if you test and your blood sugar is below 70 mg/dl, eat enough carbohydrate to raise your blood sugar to normal, remembering that 1 gram of carbohydrate raises your blood sugar about 4 points. Do not bolus for any carbs used to raise your blood sugar (or your blood sugar won't rise!).

If, like many people, you consume more carbs than needed to raise your blood sugar and find your blood sugars are always high after overtreating, this extra carbohydrate will need to be covered by a bolus as soon as your blood sugar is back to normal so that you won't have a high blood sugar later. When you eat more carbs than you need, as soon as it is safe be sure to take a bolus to match most of the extra carbs. The safer method, of course, is to not overtreat lows.

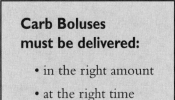

Carb Boluses must be delivered:
- in the right amount
- at the right time

In Chapter 11, you'll determine how many grams of carbohydrate are covered by each unit of bolus insulin. Once you have determined this, you can balance the bolus with the carbohydrate in your meals and have normal blood sugars afterwards.

> **Your carb boluses are correct when your blood sugar starts at a normal value before meals and ends up normal 3 1/2 hours later with Humalog or 5 hours later with Regular.**

High Blood Sugar Boluses

When your blood sugar goes high unexpectedly, a high blood sugar bolus is used to bring it down. As with balancing carbohydrates, the higher your blood sugar, the more bolus insulin is needed to bring it down to normal. Chapter 12 shows how to determine the number of points your blood sugar drops on each unit of insulin. With this information, you can create an individualized sliding scale to give you the correct bolus to lower any high blood sugar.

> **Your high blood sugar boluses are correct when they bring a high blood sugar back to normal in 3 1/2 to 4 hours on Humalog, or 5 to 6 hours on Regular.**

In setting the correct basals and boluses on a pump, or when trying to correct control problems, it is critical to know your total daily insulin dose (TDD), which will be covered in the next chapter. Luckily, most pumps record your TDD for the last few days in the pump's memory. Reviewing this information can help when control problems arise.

Workspace 8.1 Essential Numbers For Pumping

Using a pump to control your blood sugar is based on knowing certain essential numbers. As you go through the book, determining what each of these numbers is for you will make using your pump easy and effective. Write your own numbers here to keep a convenient record of them.

- Your TDD or total daily insulin dose = _____ units

- What percentage of your TDD is basal = _____%

- Basal rates =   _____ u/hr starting at _____ am/pm

    _____ u/hr starting at _____ am/pm

    _____ u/hr starting at _____ am/pm

    _____ u/hr starting at _____ am/pm

    _____ u/hr starting at _____ am/pm

    _____ u/hr starting at _____ am/pm

- Insulin to carb bolus ratio = 1 unit H per _____ grams of carb

- Point drop per one unit of insulin = 1 unit H to drop _____ points

- Point rise per gram of carb = 1 gram raises my blood sugar 4 points (4 mg/dl or 0.22 mmol)

- Unused bolus rule: on Humalog, 30% of the last bolus will be used each hour

- See Table 19.1 for how many ExCarbs you need for exercise.

"Good judgement comes from experience;
and experience, well, that comes from bad judgement.

How To Determine Your TDD

The most important thing to determine when starting on a pump, or when control problems appear, is how much insulin you need each day. This is called your total daily insulin dose (TDD), and is the first of the essential numbers to know in pumping.

Once you know your TDD, you can closely determine your basal and bolus doses. Your TDD is like true north on a compass, helping you correctly navigate your blood sugars. With an accurate TDD, you estimate your starting basal rates, insulin-to-carb ratio, and point drop ratio using Table 10.1 in the next chapter. The numbers in this book are suggestions based on clinical experience; they must always be verified by your health care team and tested for accuracy.

Although relatively steady from day to day, your TDD is not a fixed number. It will vary slightly day to day with changes in activity and carbohydrate intake. It may also vary gradually over time from factors like weight gain or loss, stress, and the seasons. Other factors, like weekend gardening, running a marathon, or monthly menses for women, may necessitate a rapid change in your TDD. Once you know your "standard" TDD, it becomes much easier to adjust for changes in lifestyle or metabolism.

In this chapter we'll show you

- How to estimate your TDD
- How to determine your basal rate(s) and boluses from your TDD

Setting Your Total Daily Dose

If you're just switching from injections to a pump, start by adding up your current TDD on injections. Realize that your daily insulin use while on injections will almost always have to be reduced. As pumping improves control, you are likely to need less insulin on a pump.[61,62] Pumps allow insulin doses to be timed to match your need precisely, which almost always requires a reduction in doses. Keep in mind that people with Type 1 diabetes often have ended up on excessive insulin doses due to numerous attempts to improve their control with injections. If you are having frequent or severe lows while on injections, this is a good sign that your injected insulin doses are too high and you will need a major reduction on a pump. Some people with Type 1 diabetes may need to cut their TDD as much as 40% to 50% in the first two to four weeks of pumping.

Unfortunately, there is no perfect way to estimate how far to reduce your injected TDD as you start on a pump. An initial method of adjusting it is suggested in the next section. Even after using this method to reduce pump doses, you may need to reduce your basals and boluses as soon as the first day or two, with additional adjustments often needed over the first 7 to 14 days.

Others who have insulin resistance, which is common in Type 2 diabetes, or have high counter-regulatory hormone levels, which is found in growing teens, may see their previous TDD of 90 units on injections drop rapidly to 45 or 50 units a day in the first week or two of pump use. On the other hand, someone who has been in very good control on multiple daily injections may find their TDD needs drop only slightly on a pump.

Occasionally, the TDD may not need to be reduced at all when starting on a pump. Examples of this would be a person who on injections was running consistently high blood sugars with no lows, a teen with excess growth hormone, or a child who has recently gained weight and needs higher insulin doses for normal growth.

How To Estimate Your TDD When Switching From Injections

Your TDD can be estimated in two ways. The first way is to simply add up how much insulin you are currently using each day. The second way is based on your weight and assumes you have a normal sensitivity to insulin. These two estimates are then compared to provide a starting TDD as you switch from injections to a pump. Use Workspace 9.1 to determine your starting TDD, using the following steps:

A. Using Part A in Workspace 9.1, add up your typical insulin doses of both the long-acting and short-acting insulin you use each day. This is your **Current TDD** or "**A**" and will provide an estimate of your new pump TDD based on your current insulin doses. Do not include extra insulin you may use to lower high blood sugars, even though this can provide additional insight into how much extra insulin you might need per day.

B. Next divide your weight in pounds by 4 (or, if you weigh in kilograms, divide your kilogram weight by 1.8). This is your **Expected TDD** or "**B**" and is an estimate of your TDD that is based on an average sensitivity to insulin for a person of your weight. The numbers are worked out for you in Table 9.1 on page 86.

Workspace 9.1 Estimate Your Starting Total Daily Dose (TDD) On A Pump

A. Determine Your Current TDD On Injections

Add up all your normal insulin doses given in 24 hours:

Breakfast: ___ u H/R + ___ u L/N/UL = ___ units

Lunch: ___ u H/R + ___ u L/N/UL = ___ units

Dinner: ___ u H/R + ___ u L/N/UL = ___ units

Bedtime: ___ u H/R + ___ u L/N/UL = ___ units

My **Current TDD** = ___ units/day (A)

Place A in Step 1 to the right

B. Then calculate your **Expected TDD** for someone of your weight (see Table 9.1):

Your weight (lbs.) divided by 4 = ___ units/day (B)

Place B in Step 2 to the right, then proceed with Step 3.

Step 1: Current TDD (A) = ___ units/day

Step 2: Expected TDD (B) = ___ units/day

Step 3: Average the numbers from Step 1 and Step 2:

Average of A and B = ___ units/day (C)

Step 4: Pick smaller number from A and C Then multiply it by 90% to get your Starting TDD:

Smaller of A and C = ___ units/day

X 0.9
_____

My **Starting TDD** = ___ units/day

C. Then use Steps 1-4 in the box to find "**C**". To get your new TDD on the pump, use 90% of the number **C** (i.e., multiply C by 0.9). This is your **Starting TDD on a pump**.

Some pump guidelines suggest that the TDD on injections should be reduced automatically by 25%. This reduction may or may not be appropriate for you, but using the method in Workspace 9.1 usually gives a close estimate of your starting TDD on a pump (It may underestimate insulin need in Type 2s who are insulin resistant). Your physician will give you your actual starting TDD, basal rates and bolus ratios.

How To Estimate Your TDD When Already On A Pump

Almost all pumps have memory, and one convenient piece of information is a history of your TDD for the last five days or more. This is very helpful if you are already on a pump but having control problems. By knowing your current TDD, you can quickly adjust this TDD as needed to correct unwanted patterns of high or low blood sugars. Refer to Table 14.1 for help on how to adjust your TDD. Once your TDD is adjusted, take this new TDD and find your basal rates and boluses using Table 10.1.

Use Your TDD To Determine Basals And Boluses

Your TDD now can be used to estimate your basal rates and boluses. In the next chapter, you will use Workspace 9.1 and Table 10.1 or 10.2, to fill in Workspace 10.1 on page 94 to determine your starting basal rate, insulin to carbohydrate ratio for carb boluses, and point drop for high blood sugar boluses. Be aware that the starting basal rate (and boluses) may need to be reduced soon after starting on a pump, especially if your blood sugar control was previously poor. The better blood sugar control seen on a pump will lessen insulin resistance and therefore lower your need for insulin.[14,63] Testing this starting basal rate(s) is covered in the next chapter.

If you are already on a pump, use these suggested basals and boluses to evaluate your current basal and bolus settings. Your TDD usually needs to be adjusted when life changes occur that impact your glucose control and insulin need. See Chapter 14 for when to adjust your TDD, basals and boluses. Anytime your life changes in certain ways, your insulin need and TDD are likely to change as well.

What if you use more or less insulin than estimated by Table 10.1? If your weight is above your ideal body weight, you eat a high fat diet, exercise only at your desk, have been in poor control for some time, or produce more hormones that block insulin than the average person, you will need more insulin. If you're a teenager with high hormone levels aiding your growth, you will need much more insulin. If you are thin, exercise regularly, or eat a very healthy diet, you may need less. Your physician/health care team's familiarity with these factors allows them to help you make accurate estimates of your basal and bolus requirements.

Table 9.1 TDD Estimated From Weight

If your wt in lbs. is:	or in kgs. is:	Your expected TDD is:
80 lbs	36 kgs	20 u
90 lbs	41 kgs	22.5 u
100 lbs	45 kgs	25 u
110 lbs	50 kgs	27.5 u
120 lbs	55 kgs	30 u
130 lbs	59 kgs	32.5 u
140 lbs	64 kgs	35 u
150 lbs	68 kgs	37.5 u
160 lbs	73 kgs	40 u
170 lbs	77 kgs	42.5 u
180 lbs	82 kgs	45 u
190 lbs	86 kgs	47.5 u
200 lbs	91 kgs	50 u
210 lbs	95 kgs	52.5 u
220 lbs	100 kgs	55 u
230 lbs	105 kgs	57.5 u
240 lbs	109 kgs	60 u
250 lbs	114 kgs	62.5 u

For safety's sake, always use the smallest TDD that seems likely to control your blood sugar. Ask your physician/health care team for assistance with these adjustments. Their experience and feedback can speed your path to better control.

Example Of Using Workspace 9.1 And Table 10.1

As an example of estimating starting basal rates, Frances weighs 160 pounds and is close to her ideal body weight. From Table 9.1, her TDD based on weight is 40 units. While on injections she has had good control taking 7 Humalog and 32 NPH before breakfast, and 9 Humalog and 12 NPH before dinner, for a TDD of 60 units. Estimating her TDD in 4 easy steps on page 85, Frances put 40 units in Step 1, 60 units in Step 2, then averaged these two values as 50 units in Step 3. Then in Step 4 she uses 90% of the 50 unit average from Step 3 to get 45 units as her TDD to start her pump.

Frances started on a single basal rate for simplicity with 50% as basal insulin and 50% as boluses. Using Table 10.1, she found her average basal rate would be approximately 0.94 u/hr, and rounded this to 0.9 units an hour. She will now test this single basal rate to see how it works, with the possibility of changing her basal rate, introducing multiple basals, and changing the percentage of her TDD given as basal.

> ### What You Need For Great Pump Control
>
> 1. Your total daily insulin dose (TDD)---the most critical information for control
>
> 2. 45 to 60% of your TDD given as basal insulin
>
> 3. 40 to 55% of your TDD given as carb boluses
>
> 4. An accurate high blood sugar bolus scale
>
> 5. ExCarbs when you exercise

The most important thing isn't a thing.

Linda Elerbee

CHAPTER 10

Setting And Testing Your Basal Rates

This chapter provides

- Sample basal rate patterns
- How to set up insulin doses using a single or multiple basals
- How to choose and test your basal rates

Setting and testing basal rates is easier when you use Humalog. With Regular, it is necessary to stop eating, take no boluses and wait for at least 5 or 6 hours before the last bolus of insulin has cleared the system. When the last bolus is no longer affecting the blood sugar, the user can begin the basal test to determine if the basal rates are properly set.

Humalog boluses clear faster than Regular. Basal testing can start 3.5 to 4 hours after the last bolus. This allows convenient basal testing without the need to go without food for extended periods. If a bolus has been taken at 7 a.m. for breakfast, basal testing can start at 10:30 a.m. or 11 a.m. On Humalog, only lunch needs to be skipped to test the afternoon basal rates.

A Single Basal Rate

A constant basal rate is the simplest way for many pumpers to start. This will satisfy insulin needs in 30% of those who go on pumps and provide a close match for

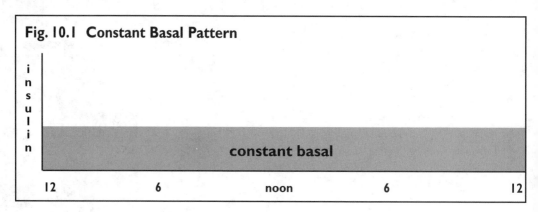

Fig. 10.1 Constant Basal Pattern

insulin

constant basal

12   6   noon   6   12

another 30%. A single rate works well for people who have Type 1 diabetes and are in good control but have little or no Dawn Phenomenon.

A constant basal rate is a good choice if you are new to pumping and prefer a simple, straightforward approach. It is also a good choice as a fresh starting point if you have been on a pump for awhile, but are having control problems. Give 50% of your TDD in equal units per hour around the clock as shown in the Constant Basal Pattern in Fig. 10.1. The gray area in Fig. 10.1 shows this basal as a straight line indicating the infusion of insulin at a constant level through the entire day.

With the use of a continuous blood sugar monitor, you can very quickly see if the constant basal rate keeps your blood sugar level. If the blood sugar begins to rise or fall at a certain time, discuss with your physician or health care team raising or lowering the basal rate beginning 3 hours earlier. Since many pumpers need more than a single basal, do not be surprised if you need to make an adjustment.

Table 10.1 gives estimated average hourly basal need based on TDD. In other words, if a person has a TDD of 24 units and wants to use 50% of the TDD as a single basal rate around the clock, she looks at Table 10.1 to find that her basal is 0.5 units/hour. This basal rate comes from taking half of 24 as the basal, then dividing by 24 hours.

See Table 10.1 for a complete breakdown of basal rates and boluses using 50% of the TDD as basal. Refer to Table 10.2 for basal rate values that make up 45%, 50% and 60% of the TDD. When basal rates make up 60% of the TDD, this may necessitate a slight reduction in the size of boluses for carbs and high blood sugars.

Whatever your starting rate or rates, it is critical that you test these settings in the first few days on your pump and then periodically retest afterwards. You may not discover the best pattern for you until you've tested and adjusted your basals several times with the help of your physician and health care team.

Multiple Basal Rates

A basal pattern designed to offset the Dawn Phenomenon and extra calorie intake at dinner when more insulin is commonly needed is called the Bicyclic Basal Pattern.

This pattern has a higher basal rate in the early morning hours to offset the Dawn Phenomenon. Around 70% to 90% of Type 1s with some Dawn Phenomenon plus most people with Type 2 diabetes need a higher basal during the early morning hours. This rate also has a higher rate during the dinner hours when carb and calorie intake is usually highest. Many people eat most of their carbs late in the day. They could balance the extra insulin needed around dinner time with carb boluses, but better control usually results when the basal is raised slightly to cover part of this need and the rest is covered by smaller carb boluses.

Lower rates are used during the night from about 8 p.m. to 2 a.m. when sensitivity to insulin is naturally at its highest, and also from about 10 a.m. to 4 p.m. when sensitivity is high because people are more active. If you have an increased need during the early morning hours and around dinner time, and are capable of handling complexity from the beginning, start with the Bicyclic Basal Pattern.

To set up the Bicyclic Basal Pattern for normal sleep hours, the lower basal is used from about 2 hours before bedtime until 3 to 4 hours after going to sleep, and again from around 10 a.m. until 4 p.m.

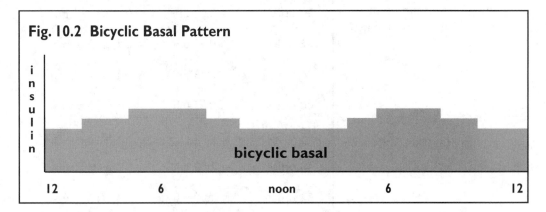

Fig. 10.2 Bicyclic Basal Pattern

People who have the Dawn Phenomenon often raise their basal rate starting between 2 a.m. and 3 a.m. (Humalog) or 1 a.m. and 3 a.m. (Regular), and then lower it between 9 a.m. and 11 a.m. The rise in the blood sugar starting at about 3 a.m. or 4 a.m. is caused by an increased release of growth hormone, which blocks the action of insulin.[64] This blockage triggers the liver to release glucose. If the insulin level is kept high, the liver won't release glucose.

A high basal rate is used during the early morning/breakfast period and again through dinner. Make sure the higher rate causes the blood sugar to drop no more than 30 mg/dl (1.7 mmol) over a 5 hour period during the day, and no more than 30 mg/dl over eight hours of sleep. When you set basals slightly higher during breakfast and dinner, set boluses for all meals slightly lower. A typical basal profile for someone who goes to sleep at 10 p.m. and rises at 6 a.m. is shown in Fig. 10.2.

In this table, you can find the numbers critical for obtaining excellent blood sugar control on a pump. Once you know your TDD from Workspace 9.1, come here to find your estimated basal rates and boluses. The average basal rates are averaged to two decimal points to provide as accurate an estimate as possible, even though an insulin pump is not this accurate.

Table 10.1 Estimated Starting Basal Rates And Boluses

For this TDD:	At 50% Basal, Avg. Basal is:	Carb Boluses:	High BG Boluses:
16 units	0.33 u/h	1 u/31 grams	1 H/112 pt. drop
18 units	0.38 u/h	1 u/28 grams	1 H/100 pt. drop
20 units	0.42 u/h	1 u/25 grams	1 H/90 pt. drop
22 units	0.46 u/h	1 u/23 grams	1 H/82 pt. drop
24 units	0.50 u/h	1 u/21 grams	1 H/75 pt. drop
26 units	0.54 u/h	1 u/19 grams	1 H/69 pt. drop
28 units	0.58 u/h	1 u/18 grams	1 H/64 pt. drop
30 units	0.62 u/h	1 u/17 grams	1 H/60 pt. drop
32 units	0.67 u/h	1 u/15 grams	1 H/56 pt. drop
36 units	0.75 u/h	1 u/14 grams	1 H/50 pt. drop
40 units	0.83 u/h	1 u/12 grams	1 H/45 pt. drop
44 units	0.92 u/h	1 u/11 grams	1 H/41 pt. drop
48 units	1.00 u/h	1 u/10 grams	1 H/38 pt. drop
52 units	1.08 u/h	1 u/10 grams	1 H/35 pt. drop
56 units	1.16 u/h	1 u/9 grams	1 H/32 pt. drop
60 units	1.25 u/h	1 u/8 grams	1 H/30 pt. drop
65 units	1.35 u/h	1 u/8 grams	1 H/28 pt. drop
70 units	1.46 u/h	1 u/7 grams	1 H/26 pt. drop
75 units	1.56 u/h	1 u/7 grams	1 H/24 pt. drop
80 units	1.67 u/h	1 u/6 grams	1 H/22 pt. drop
90 units	1.88 u/h	1 u/6 grams	1 H/20 pt. drop
100 units	2.08 u/h	1 u/5 grams	1 H/18 pt. drop

This table provides a handy way to determine your average basal rate when using 45%, 50%, or 60% of your TDD as basal insulin delivery. The average basal rates are averaged to two decimal points to provide as accurate an estimate as possible, even though an insulin pump is not this accurate.

Table 10.2 What Your Average Basal Rate Will Be As 45%, 50% or 60% Of TDD			
For this TDD:	**At 45% Basal, Avg. Basal is:**	**At 50% Basal, Avg. Basal is:**	**At 60% Basal, Avg. Basal is:**
16 units	0.30 u/h	0.33 u/h	0.40 u/h
18 units	0.34 u/h	0.38 u/h	0.45 u/h
20 units	0.38 u/h	0.42 u/h	0.50 u/h
22 units	0.41 u/h	0.46 u/h	0.55 u/h
24 units	0.45 u/h	0.50 u/h	0.60 u/h
26 units	0.49 u/h	0.54 u/h	0.65 u/h
28 units	0.52 u/h	0.58 u/h	0.70 u/h
30 units	0.56 u/h	0.62 u/h	0.75 u/h
32 units	0.60 u/h	0.67 u/h	0.80 u/h
36 units	0.68 u/h	0.75 u/h	0.90 u/h
40 units	0.75 u/h	0.83 u/h	1.00 u/h
44 units	0.82 u/h	0.92 u/h	1.10 u/h
48 units	0.90 u/h	1.00 u/h	1.20 u/h
52 units	0.98 u/h	1.08 u/h	1.30 u/h
56 units	1.05 u/h	1.16 u/h	1.40 u/h
60 units	1.12 u/h	1.25 u/h	1.50 u/h
65 units	1.35 u/h	1.35 u/h	1.62 u/h
70 units	1.46 u/h	1.46 u/h	1.75 u/h
75 units	1.56 u/h	1.56 u/h	1.88 u/h
80 units	1.67 u/h	1.67 u/h	2.00 u/h
90 units	1.88 u/h	1.88 u/h	2.25 u/h
100 units	2.08 u/h	2.08 u/h	2.50 u/h

Why raise the basal rate so long before the blood sugar begins to rise? Because it takes 60 to 120 minutes on Humalog or 90 to 180 minutes on Regular for the blood insulin level to begin to rise after the basal rate has been raised. Since basal rates are changed by only 0.1 or 0.2 units at a time, a lead time of 3 to 6 hours is needed for the basal rate to accumulate the effect needed to keep blood sugars from rising or falling. Better blood sugar control will result from a small basal rate increase at 1 a.m. or 2 a.m. than from a larger one at 3 a.m. or 4 a.m., after the liver has already begun producing glucose.

Before attempting to cover the Dawn Phenomenon, discuss this increased night basal rate carefully with your physician/health care team. Extra caution is required when raising nighttime basal rates due to the increased risk for low blood sugars during the night. Never assume you have a Dawn Phenomenon without confirmation.

The Bicyclic Basal Pattern also raises the basal in the late afternoon because many people eat most of their daily food about two hours later. The lower rate is given from 9 or 10 p.m. until 2 or 3 a.m., and from about 10 a.m. to 4 p.m. The basal is raised slightly at other times.

Workspace 10.1 Estimate Your Starting Basal Rates And Boluses

A. With your new **Starting Pump TDD** from Step 4 in Workspace 9.1, use Table 10.1 or 10.2 to find your **average basal rate** for the day. If you will be using multiple basals, distribute your average basal through the day as directed by your physician in Step 2 on the right.

B. Next find your **insulin-to-carb ratio**, using Table 10.1 or 10.2. Place this value in Step 3.

C. Again using Table 10.1 or 10.2, find your **point drop per unit** to set up high BG boluses. Place this value in Step 4.

Step 1: Get your TTD calculated in Step 4 of Workspace 9.1:

My Starting TDD = _____ units/day

Step 2: My average basal rate for the day = _____ unit/hour as a single rate, or as these multiple basals:

_12_ am	_____ u/hr
_____ am/pm	_____ u/hr
_____ am/pm	_____ u/hr
_____ am/pm	_____ u/hr
_____ am/pm	_____ u/hr
_____ am/pm	_____ u/hr
_____ am/pm	_____ u/hr

Step 3: My insulin-to-carb ratio is:

1 unit of Humalog
for each _____ grams of carbohydrate

Step 4: My blood sugar drops
_____ mg/dl per unit of Humalog

A person on the Bicyclic Basal Pattern uses at least two different basal rates, but may use various rates through a 24-hour period. Keep in mind that these rates will not vary greatly from one another for the vast majority of people. When possible, make only one adjustment at a time.

With your physician's help, choose a basal pattern and then test it. As mentioned above, the simplest pattern would be a Constant Basal Pattern for the entire day, but the Bicyclic Basal Pattern offers better control to many pumpers.

What Percentage Of Your TDD Should Be Basal?

Research studies show that the nondiabetic individual uses about 45% of the body's total daily insulin production as basal insulin. Some people on a pump do well with their basal at 45% of TDD, but others do better at 50% or even 60%. Someone who exercises a lot may need the lower percent of TDD for the basal rate.

A basal rate higher than 50% works better for many other people because it cuts down on post-meal spiking. With a slightly higher basal rate, less insulin is given as boluses and blood sugar control improves with fewer ups and downs.

A person who snacks or grazes

> **Control Problems?**
>
> Check your basal rates first. A good basal rate lets you keep your blood sugar normal when you skip meals.
>
> Quick Check: Do your basal rates make up 45% to 60% of your TDD?

during part of the day may want a larger percentage of the TDD as basal. People with a strong Dawn Phenomenon or with significant insulin resistance, may find they need as much as 60% of their TDD as basal. Teens with high levels of hormones especially benefit from a basal that is 60% of TDD. Because this pattern is based on 60% of the TDD, meal boluses are slightly lower. Many clinicians suggest starting at 50% of the TDD as basal, and adjusting as necessary.

Preventing Nighttime And Afternoon Lows

Whether you start with a Constant Basal Pattern or the Bicyclic Basal Pattern, you may need slight adjustments to your basal pattern to prevent nighttime or afternoon lows. The lowest blood sugar of the day for people with diabetes is most likely to occur around 2 a.m. In one study of people on both conventional injections and multiple daily injections, researchers found that people with Type 1 diabetes had a low blood sugar every fourth night on average.[65] Nighttime lows are more common in Type 1 diabetes, but they also occur in those with Type 2 diabetes.

People are more prone to lows in the middle of the night because the body is most sensitive to insulin between midnight and 3 a.m. The liver increases its glucose production 2 to 4 hours before waking. If lows happen in the middle of the night, the basal rate needs to be reduced by 9 p.m. or 10 p.m. to prevent the drop.

Lifestyle changes that can contribute to night lows include any extra exercise or activity during the day; this can lower blood sugars for the next 24 to 36 hours. This problem can be avoided by eating extra free carbohydrate at bedtime following an unusually active day. Overtreating a high bedtime blood sugar can also create a night low.

Waking up in the middle of the night shaking and sweating is not a pleasant experience. This middle-of-the-night drop in the blood sugar usually means that the blood insulin level needs to be lowered, often between the hours of 10 p.m. and 2 a.m. To do this, lower your basal rate at least 2 to 3 hours before 10 p.m. (at 7 or 8 p.m.)

Often pumpers require less insulin in the middle of the night to avoid lows, but they also need more insulin before waking to prevent their blood sugar from rising

> ### Why Patterns Are More Important Than Having A "Normal" Fasting Number
>
> Gwenn had just started on her pump. She was thrilled that her blood sugars were finally normal as she woke up on one of her first mornings on the pump. She thought her pump settings were perfect.
>
> However, her physician did not agree. He noticed a disturbing drop in her blood sugars during the night. Although Gwenn's blood sugar was 87 mg/dl (4.8 mmol), her 1 a.m. reading earlier that night had been 181 mg/dl (10 mmol). She did not bolus for this high reading at 1 a.m., but her blood sugar dropped over 90 points (5 mmol) by dawn anyway. Imagine if Gwenn's reading had been 90 mg/dl at 1 a.m.! She and her physician decided to reduce her nighttime basal rates immediately, even without testing for another night.

because of a Dawn Phenomenon. This pattern is often seen in Type 1 diabetes, while in Type 2 diabetes there is an increased need for insulin in the early morning hours to stop the liver from producing excess glucose because of insulin resistance. In Type 1, the basal rate with Humalog may need to be reduced by 9 or 10 p.m., then raised higher than the usual daytime level at 1 a.m. to 3 a.m. In Type 2 diabetes when insulin resistance is present, only the basal rate increase at 1 a.m. to 3 a.m. applies. Later, at 9 a.m. to 11 a.m., the basal rate is lowered back to normal in both instances.

If you think you are having nighttime lows, test at 2 a.m. for a few nights. If insulin reactions are occurring in the middle of the night, lower your basal rate at 9 or 10 p.m., with a return to normal between 1 a.m. and 3 a.m. Using Regular insulin increases the risk for afternoon and nighttime low blood sugars because of an overlapping buildup from carb boluses due to Regular's long action time.

Another common problem for many people is needing less insulin in the afternoon. These individuals are often physically active. They will get afternoon lows if an excess of insulin has built up in the blood from the boluses given for breakfast and lunch, especially if Regular is used. This is more common in Type 1 diabetes but can occur in either type.

To avoid afternoon lows, reduce your bolus for lunch carbohydrates or reduce the basal rate through the afternoon. A basal reduction may be needed at 10 a.m. or 11 a.m. with Regular to prevent lows at 4 p.m., while for Humalog a reduction by 11 a.m. or noon would work.

Because of the precision and flexibility of insulin delivery with a pump, adjusting the rate for changing insulin need during the day is easy. Some pumpers, particularly those who exercise strenuously or for prolonged periods, find they benefit from 3 to 6 different basal rates each day to ensure insulin levels that are lower during and after exercise. Temporary basal rate reductions also are convenient for exercise.

With experience, you will learn to make these changes as needed. Be sure to consult with your physician/health care team if you are uncertain what your results mean or if you suspect that you need more than one basal rate during the day. The basal rate tests below will clarify what your own basal insulin needs are.

Correct Basal Rates are Critical For Blood Sugar Control.

How To Test Your Basal Rates

In this chapter, you'll take your estimated starting basal rate(s) from Workspace 10.1 and test it for accuracy. If you are just starting on an insulin pump, the first test of your basal rates has to be delayed until the last injection of long-acting insulin is no longer lowering your blood sugar. Basal testing cannot begin until 24 hours after the last injection of Lente or NPH or 36 hours after the last injection of Ultralente or Lantus (glargine).

Initial basal rate estimates are tested in the first 3 to 4 days of pump use. Basal rates are retested any time that signs indicate a need for a higher or lower rate. A basal rate that is too high is suggested by frequent lows, by a drop in the blood sugar when a meal is skipped, or by weight gain over time due to increased eating to compensate for lows. A basal rate that is too low is suggested by frequent highs, by a rise in the blood sugar when a meal is skipped, or by the need for frequent corrections with high blood sugar boluses.

Blood sugars need to be monitored frequently while testing your basal rates. A continuous monitoring device will quickly reveal if your basal rates are keeping your blood sugar level, and built-in alarms help you avoid low blood sugars. The goal is to find a basal rate that will keep the blood sugar flat and level or cause it to fall only slightly when no food is eaten. Basal testing is broken into an overnight and three daytime segments during the day for convenience. Pumpers who work odd hours, a nightshift, or varied shifts will need to adjust testing times for their schedules.

Test The Night Basal Rate

Basal rates are tested first before boluses. The overnight basal is usually tested first since it is so important for preventing nighttime reactions and allows you to wake up with a normal reading. Tests are repeated until desirable basal results are obtained on two or more occasions. Once the night basal rate is correctly set, it's easy to wake up with a normal reading.

Not only do you experience a full night of sound sleep, but your day starts better when you wake up with a normal blood sugar. Waking up during the night in the middle of an insulin reaction or thirsty and tired from a high blood sugar doesn't promote sound sleep. Having a steady blood sugar in a desirable range through the night is the first step to having normal readings through the day.

An accurate night basal rate lets you

- go to bed with a normal blood sugar, eat little or no bedtime snack, and wake up with a normal blood sugar in the morning
- safely correct a high bedtime blood sugar and wake up with a normal reading in the morning
- rest peacefully. You, your spouse, parents, children, friends, roommates, and physician/health care team will all sleep better knowing you're unlikely to have a reaction during the night

Don't try this test following a day in which you've had a major insulin reaction, major emotional stress, or unusually strenuous exercise. Major insulin reactions and excessive stress cause the release of stress hormones into the bloodstream that raise blood sugar levels for the next few hours. Strenuous exercise can have just the opposite effect by enhancing insulin's action and lowering the blood sugar for several hours. Occurrences like these in the hours before your test can distort your results.

Directions for basal testing can be found in Table 10.3 on page 101. Test the blood sugar near bedtime at least 3.5 hours following the last bolus of Humalog. If this reading is between 100 and 150 mg/dl (5.6 to 8.3 mmol) or 120 to 180 mg/dl (6.7 to 10 mmol) may be preferred for those with hypoglycemia unawareness, proceed to test the basal rate. This allows room for the blood sugar to fall if the basal rate is set too high. Once the basal rate is correctly set, ideal blood sugars can be achieved and maintained safely.

Do not eat anything before bed and do not take a bolus. If your blood sugar is 70 to 100 mg/dl (3.9 to 5.6 mmol), you can eat 15 to 20 grams of glucose tabs or other quick carbs and retest in another 30 minutes to start your night basal test.

Test your blood sugar at 2 a.m. to determine if it is rising or dropping. The goal for the middle of the night test is for blood sugars to stay at the same level, or to have dropped no more than 20 points from the bedtime reading. On waking, if the blood sugar has remained level or dropped no farther than 30 points from the bedtime reading, the basal settings are appropriate for keeping the blood sugar level overnight.

Don't forget the 2 a.m. test! This middle-of-the-night test is critical for catching nighttime lows, and for determining whether more than one basal rate is needed during the night and whether and when the night basal rate needs to be increased or

Example: Testing And Setting The Night Basal

Jeremy is 28 years old and was estimated to need a TDD of 40 units when he started on his pump. For simplicity, he was started on a constant basal of 0.8 u/hr around the clock. On his first overnight basal test, he got these results:

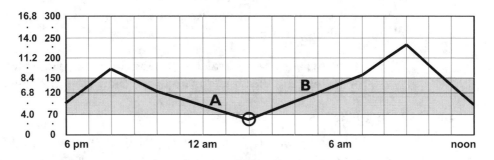

His results show a drop in his blood sugar between 10 p.m. and 2 a.m.(A), an insulin reaction at 2 a.m., followed by a rising blood sugar from 2 a.m. to 8 a.m. (B) Because his physician believes in stopping lows first, they decided to lower his overnight basal to 0.7 u/hr between 8 p.m. and 8 a.m. to avoid low blood sugars in the middle of the night. He got this result when he tested the new basal rate:

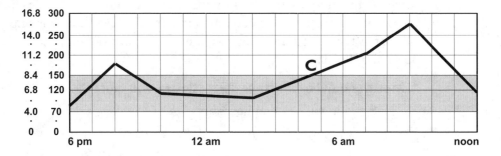

On 0.7 u/hr, Jeremy was able to stop the middle of the night low blood sugar, but now has a large rise in his blood sugar between 2 a.m. and 7 a.m. (C), probably due to a Dawn Phenomenon. After one basal increase, retesting, and a second increase in the morning basal, he and his physician finally settled on a rate of 0.7 u/hr between 8 p.m. and 1 a.m. and a rate of 0.9 u/hr between 1 a.m. and 9 a.m. with these results:

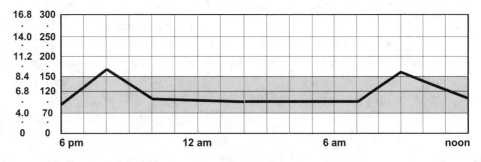

decreased. If you are below 70 mg/dl (3.9 mmol) at the 2 a.m. test, eat a 15 gram snack and reduce the basal rate between 8, 9, or 10 p.m. until 2 a.m. for the next test.

From your blood sugar test results, adjust your basal rates. Raise or lower the basal rate as instructed until the basal rate keeps your blood sugar relatively flat on at least two consecutive tests on different nights. Always check with physician/health care team if you have any doubts about your doses, about how to interpret the readings or whether to change the timing or level of your basal rate.

The correct night basal rate keeps the blood sugar from rising or lowers the blood sugar no more than 30 points overnight.

Test The Day Basal Rates

When testing your day basal rates (see Table 10.3) you want nothing to interfere with your blood sugars, like a recent meal, a residual bolus of insulin, prolonged exercise that day, unusual stress, or the aftermath of a major insulin reaction. You'll want to start these tests either when you get up in the morning or when at least 3.5 hours have passed since your last Humalog bolus and 3 hours after your last food. This ensures that only the basal rate will be affecting the blood sugars.

Testing the day basal rate is done in three parts for convenience and to avoid changes in sensitivity that occur with longer periods of fasting. Testing in three segments allows most meals to be eaten on test days even though eating may be delayed. Each test is repeated until the basal works well on two consecutive tests during that period of the day.

Once the day basal rate is correctly set, you can

- skip meals when necessary
- eat meals late without the worry of a reaction
- bolus precisely for carbohydrates and high blood sugars

Skipping meals is required to test your basal rates. People who have had diabetes for awhile often have reservations about skipping meals for testing or any other reason. Some simply find it difficult to imagine going a few hours without food, but the human body is amazingly adaptive and will survive this ordeal. Some object: "They've always told me to eat when I take any insulin," but the beauty of a pump is that a correct basal rate eliminates the need to eat.

A few hours of fasting is a small price to pay for a correctly set basal rate since this is usually the most important step toward having normal blood sugars. If you are concerned about having a reaction on your current basal rate, check your blood sugar more often, and consult with your physician/health care team about doing your test with a lower basal rate.

The blood sugar at the start of the test is ideally between 100 and 150 mg/dl (5.6 to 8.3 mmol). The first part starts when you wake in the morning and ends at noon.

Table 10.3 How To Test Your Basal Rates

Test	Preparation	BG Tests	What To Do With Test Results
Night Basal	Start at least 3.5 hours after your last Humalog bolus, when your bedtime blood sugar is between 100 mg/dl and 150 mg/dl (5.6 to 8.3 mmol).	Test at bedtime, at 2 AM, and on waking	A good basal rate will keep your blood sugar level or make it fall no more than 30 points during 8 hrs. of sleep. If your blood sugar rises, raise your basal rate slightly and retest. If it falls over 30 points, reduce the basal rate and retest. With a good result, retest to verify.
Day Basal, 1st part	Start when your blood sugar is between 100 mg/dl and 150 mg/dl (5.6 to 8.3 mmol) on waking. Skip breakfast and breakfast bolus, and begin test.	Test at start, and every hour for 5 hrs.	A good basal rate will keep your blood sugar level or make it fall no more than 30 points during 5 hrs. of fasting. If your blood sugar rises, raise your basal rate slightly and retest. If it falls over 30 points, reduce the basal rate and retest. With a good result, retest to verify.
Day Basal, 2nd part	Start when your blood sugar is between 100 mg/dl and 150 mg/dl (5.6 to 8.3 mmol) before lunch. Skip lunch and lunch bolus, and begin test.	Test at start, and every hour for 5 hrs	Same
Day Basal, 3rd part	Start when your blood sugar is between 100 mg/dl and 150 mg/dl (5.6 to 8.3 mmol) before dinner. Skip dinner and dinner bolus, and begin test.	Test at start, and every hour for 5 hrs	Same

End your test and eat at any time your blood sugar goes low.
Take a bolus and end test if your blood sugar goes above 180 mg/dl.
Timing for tests may vary depending on your normal schedule.

The second part of the test covers the lunch hour and into the afternoon. During this part, eat breakfast, skip lunch and afternoon snacks, and then eat dinner. In the third test, eat breakfast and lunch, but fast after lunch until bedtime. Eat a late dinner just before bedtime if you wish.

Summary

First Part of Day Test

The first part of the day basal test starts when you wake in the morning and ends at lunch. If your night basal showed that a single basal rate worked well for you all night, the day basal rate is likely to be identical or very similar to this night rate. However, if your basal rate needed to be increased in the early morning hours for a Dawn Phenomenon, one of the first things you need to determine is when after breakfast does this higher waking rate need to be reduced.

On a day when you wake up with a blood sugar between 100 and 150 mg/dl (5.6 to 8.3 mmol), skip breakfast and your breakfast bolus. Test your blood sugar each hour or at any time you suspect your blood sugar may be high or low. A good basal rate will keep your blood sugar flat over the next 5 hours or cause it to drop no more than 30 mg/dl (1.7 mmol), say from 120 mg/dl (6.7 mmol) at 7 a.m. to 90 mg/dl at noon. Then have your lunch, unless a low blood sugar has already necessitated eating.

Do this test on a day when you expect to be at your normal level of activity, since extra work or exercise will lower the blood sugar. As in the night basal test and the tests that follow, there must be no strenuous exercise, excess stress, or a major insulin reaction in the hours preceding the test. Test this rate on another day until you get desirable results on two occasions at the same basal rates.

Second Part of Day Test

The second part starts before lunch and ends in the late afternoon on another day. After setting your morning rate, test the afternoon basal rate by skipping lunch and any afternoon snack. Since you've already found the correct basal rate for the morning, start this test with the same rate or a slightly lower rate for the middle of the day.

If you are on a Bicyclic Basal Pattern, your morning basal rate has usually been lowered slightly at about 10 a.m., and is left this way until about 4 p.m. when it is raised. Adjust these times to fit your schedule as needed. Repeat the test until you find a basal rate that gives a stable blood sugar through the afternoon.

Third Part of Day Test

The third part covers late afternoon to bedtime. Since you've already found the correct basal rate or rates for the morning and afternoon hours and also the rate for starting the night basal, the basal rate for this test should be very close to the preceding and following rates. Skip dinner and start testing. If you use a Bicyclic Basal Pattern, the dinner basal rate will be higher than later in the evening so you'll need to determine when to lower the dinner rate. Eight or nine p.m. works well for many.

Remember that when you use Humalog, the basal rate has to be reduced at least 3 to 6 hours before the blood sugar starts its fall. It must also be raised 3 to 6 hours before a rise is seen in the blood sugar. Because the extra insulin coming from a higher basal rate continues to work for 3 hours after the rate is lowered, the basal rate must be adjusted downward long before the blood sugar actually might start to drop.

A good basal principle is to make changes early and small.

Tips On Basal Testing

• Always consult with your physician/health care team to select your starting basal rate(s).

• Test and set your night basal first, since this will let you wake up with a normal blood sugar and reduce the risk of nighttime lows.

• For the first part of the day test, eat no breakfast. For the second part of the day, eat no lunch. For the third part of the day, eat no dinner until close to bedtime. Of course, eat anytime a low blood sugar requires it and discontinue the test.

• Test your blood sugar more often if you believe it may drop.

• If your blood sugar drops below 70 mg/dl (3.9 mmol), have at least 15 grams of carbohydrate and end the test. Discuss lowering your basal rate with your physician/health care team. If the drop in blood sugar is rapid, a major decrease in the basal rate is needed. If the drop occurs slowly, a small decrease is needed.

• If your blood sugar rises above 200 mg/dl (11 mmol), take a bolus to correct the high blood sugar and end the test. Discuss raising your basal rate with your physician/health care team. If your blood sugar rises rapidly, a major increase in the basal rate probably is needed. If the rise occurs slowly, a small increase may do the trick.

A good basal rate keeps your blood sugar level, or allows it to fall no more than 30 points during any test period.

With experience, you will be testing and making changes as needed. Be sure to consult with your physician/health care team if you are uncertain what your test results mean.

Never change your basal rate based on one day's tests unless the rate is unquestionably incorrect. Also, never assume a rate is correct after one day's test. Test twice to confirm.

Tips On Basal Rates

• Most people benefit from having more than one basal rate a day. If you require several basal rates, these rates should not vary greatly from each other.

- The best basal rate is one that causes the blood sugar to stay constant or to drop slightly over several hours while not eating.

- Carbohydrate may be needed when the bedtime blood sugar is less than 100 mg/dl (5.6 mmol).

- With Humalog, change a basal rate 3 to 6 hours before the blood sugar begins its rise or fall.

- Control of a Dawn Phenomenon often is better if the basal rate is raised by 0.1 to 0.2 u/hr at 1 a.m. or 2 a.m. than by a larger increase at 3 a.m. or 4 a.m.

Signs your basal rate is too high:

- your blood sugar drops when you skip a meal.
- you have frequent lows in the early morning or before breakfast.
- you have frequent lows during the day.

Signs your basal rate is too low:

- your blood sugar rises when you skip a meal.
- you have frequent high blood sugars.
- you have frequent need for high blood sugar boluses to bring down high blood sugars.

Other basal considerations:

- Change your basal rate in small increments (usually by 0.1 unit an hour) long before the need occurs. For instance, if low blood sugars occur on waking, lower the basal rates as early as midnight or 10 p.m. to prevent the waking low.

- Generally your basal rates will be grouped closely together. For instance, if the highest rate is 1.1 unit/hr, you would expect your lowest rate to be no lower than 0.7 unit/hr.

- If your activity or stress level is very different on weekends, set and test a different basal profile for the weekend. Again test the overnight basal first, and then the daytime in three segments.

- Add your basals up periodically or check the basal totals on your pump to make sure they make up 45% to 60% of your TDD.

Quick Basal Rate Check: Does the daily basal insulin dose make up 45% to 60% of the total daily insulin dose?

Fall seven times, stand up eight.
Japanese proverb

Setting And Testing Your Carb Boluses

"How much insulin do I take to cover a bagel, a dish of pasta, or a bowl of fruit?" This critical question can be answered by determining how many grams of carbohydrate are present in the food you want to eat and then using your insulin-to-carb ratio to determine how many bolus units you need to cover them.

Like all insulin doses, your ratio of Humalog to carbohydrate can be determined from your TDD. When carb intake is balanced with appropriate boluses, it gives you tremendous freedom in your food choices and in the timing of your meals.

Most people require a unit of insulin for somewhere between 6 to 20 grams of carbohydrate. However, someone who is very thin or very physically active may need only one unit of Humalog for every 25 grams of carbohydrate, while a growing teen may need one unit for every 5 grams. Someone with Type 2 diabetes and severe insulin resistance may need a unit for every 2 grams.

This chapter shows:

- How to set your insulin-to-carb ratio
- How to test this ratio
- How to time carb boluses for good coverage

Setting The Insulin-To-Carb Ratio

Your Humalog (or Regular) to carb ratio is based on your TDD and can be determined from Table 10.1 or Table 11.1. Determining a starting ratio that will

105

closely estimate how many grams of carbohydrate one unit of Humalog will cover for you is as easy as looking it up in these tables.

The starting insulin-to-carb ratio is based on what we call the 500 Rule. Simply divide the number 500 by your TDD to find out how many carbs will be covered by one unit of Humalog. For example, someone whose TDD is 20 units will need one unit of Humalog for every 25 grams of carbohydrate (500/20 = 25), while someone else using 50 units a day will need one unit for every 10 grams (500/50 = 10).

The number 500 has been derived from the clinical experience of diabetes specialists over the years. Your own starting insulin-to-carb ratio should always be verified with a personal recommendation from your physician/health care team. If you have Type 2 diabetes and insulin resistance, the 500 Rule may underestimate your true insulin need. If you have Type 1, are thin and physically active, this rule may overestimate the actual insulin need.

To determine the bolus needed for a meal, first count the grams of carbohydrate you'll be eating. Carb counting, explained in Chapter 7 and Appendix A, is a simple step toward improving blood sugar control. Divide the total carbs in the meal by your insulin-to-carb ratio to get the bolus amount needed to cover it. For instance, if you take one unit for every 12 grams of carb and want to eat a 24-gram snack, you would take a 2-unit bolus.

Testing Carb Boluses

Once you have an estimate of your insulin-to-carb ratio, Workspace 11.1 on page 109 can be used to see if this ratio is correct for you. This starting estimate of your carb ratio must be tested to see if it is accurate. It is best to test your carb boluses after your basal rate(s) have been adjusted and now keep your blood sugars relatively flat.

It helps to be as consistent as possible in how much carbohydrate you eat at each meal and in the timing of meals until your insulin-to-carb ratio has been thoroughly tested. This speeds the testing process. Later, you can eat in a flexible fashion once your carb ratio has been tested and determined to be accurate.

To start a test, check your blood sugar 15 minutes before a meal. You want this reading to be between 70 and 150 mg/dl (3.9 to 8.3 mmol). Test your carb bolus only when you have had no insulin reactions in the last 4 hours. Count the grams of carbohydrate you plan to eat in the upcoming meal. Then divide the total carb count by the number of grams of carbohydrate covered by 1 unit of insulin. The resulting number gives the size of your meal bolus. For instance, if you use a unit for every 10 grams of carb and want to eat 70 grams, you would take a 7 unit bolus.

Take this about 15 minutes before the meal with Humalog or 30 minutes before with Regular. Test your blood sugar at hourly intervals after the meal. An acceptable blood sugar rise at one hour would be 40 to 80 mg/dl (2.2 to 4.4 mmol) above the starting blood sugar. If your blood sugar at one hour rises less than 40 mg/dl, your bolus may have been too large; begin testing your blood sugar every half hour to avoid a low. If your blood sugar at one hour is above 240 mg/dl (13.3 mmol), end the test and correct the high blood sugar.

A correct insulin-to-carb ratio will return your blood sugar to within 30 points (1.7 mmol) of the starting blood sugar after 3.5 hours with Humalog or after 5 hours with Regular, although these times may be delayed somewhat following high fat meals or very large boluses. If your ratio appears to be correct, repeat the test at least two more times to verify this ratio is correct for you.

Any low blood sugar you have after giving this bolus suggests your ratio needs to be changed. If a low happens only an hour or two after the bolus, this suggests a larger change in the insulin-to-carb ratio is needed, while if lows occur three or four hours later, less change is needed. For instance, if lows occur an hour or two after you eat and you are using 1 unit of Humalog for each 12 grams, try adding two or three grams to the carbohydrate next time. Now you will be using 1 unit of Humalog for each 14 or 15 grams. This gives you less insulin for the same amount of carbohydrate and makes low blood sugars less likely.

However, if the low blood sugar happens 3 or 4 hours after a Humalog bolus or 4 or 5 hours after a Regular bolus, your insulin-to-carb ratio only needs a slight adjustment. Try adding 1 to the carbohydrate number, so that instead of 1 Humalog for each 12 grams, it now becomes 1 Humalog for each 13 grams. If high blood sugars occur during testing, be more cautious and subtract only 1 from the carb ratio, i.e., 1 H for each 11 grams of carb.

With Humalog, your test is successful if your blood sugar three and a half hours after the meal is within 30 mg/dl of the starting

Table 11.1 Set Your Insulin-To-Carb Ratio With 500 Rule	
For this TDD:	Your Carb Bolus is:
16 units	1 u/31 grams
18 units	1 u28 grams
20 units	1 u/25 grams
22 units	1 u/23 grams
24 units	1 u/21 grams
26 units	1 u/19 grams
28 units	1 u/18 grams
30 units	1 u/17 grams
32 units	1 u/15 grams
36 units	1 u/14 grams
40 units	1 u/12 grams
44 units	1 u/11 grams
48 units	1 u/10 grams
52 units	1 u/10 grams
56 units	1 u/9 grams
60 units	1 u/8 grams
65 units	1 u/8 grams
70 units	1 u/7 grams
75 units	1 u/7 grams
80 units	1 u/6 grams
90 units	1 u/6 grams
100 units	1 u/5 grams

blood sugar. If you use Regular, the test taken five hours after the meal should be within 30 points of the starting blood sugar to indicate the correct bolus ratio.

Some people find that a unit of insulin may cover fewer carbohydrate grams at breakfast than at other meals. A decreased insulin sensitivity in the morning often results from production of more glucose-raising hormones, especially growth hormone, in the early morning hours. If you need a larger bolus at breakfast than at lunch or dinner for the same amount of carbohydrate, you will want to ask your doctor about raising your early morning basal rate so that you can start your day better.

If you use Regular in your pump, the insulin-to-carb ratio may need to vary slightly for different meals of the day. Boluses of Regular given early in the day for breakfast and lunch overlap during the afternoon and evening hours due to Regular's long action time.[66-] Because of Humalog's faster action and shorter duration, a bolus enters and leaves the blood faster. This reduces the problems encountered with Regular insulin caused by overlapping boluses.

If your insulin-to-carb ratio usually works for you, but you experience a high or low blood sugar after a particular meal or snack, consider:

- Did you count the carbs carefully in the meal?
- Did you take your bolus the usual number of minutes before eating?
- Did the meal have an unusually high or low glycemic index?

Another way to determine your ratio is to use a standard meal plan combined with carb counting. Here you can distribute your daily carbs, with each meal and snack having a set carbohydrate amount. If you use 50% of your TDD as basal insulin, the other 50% can be divided into your day's total carb amount. For instance, if your TDD is 50 units, and you are allowed 300 grams of carbs each day, you would take half of the 50 units, or 25 units, as your carb insulin. Dividing this into 300 grams gives you 1 unit of Humalog for each 12 grams of carbohydrate.

If your breakfast has 72 grams of carb each day, you would take a bolus of 6.0 units to cover it. Testing the carb bolus would then determine whether an adjustment

Quick Check: Do your boluses make up about half of your TDD?

If your TDD is:	Your boluses/day would be about:
20 units	10 units
25 units	12 units
30 units	15 units
35 units	17 units
40 units	20 units
50 units	25 units
60 units	30 units
70 units	35 units
80 units	40 units
90 units	45 units
100 units	50 units

Workspace 11.1 How To Test Your Humalog Insulin-To-Carbohydrate Ratio

Prepare	Make sure that your basal rates have been tested and correctly set before starting.

Use Table 10.1 or Table 11.1 and your physician's help to decide how many grams of carbohydrate are covered by one unit of Humalog. Place this value to the right.

_____ grams of carb covered by one unit of Humalog = **A**

Start	When your blood sugar is 80 to 120 mg/dl (4.4 to 6.7 mmol), and you have had no boluses and no food within the last 3.5 hours and no recent insulin reactions.

Do The Math

How many grams of carbohydrate will you eat?   _____ grams of carb = **B**

Divide the grams of carb you will eat (**B**) by how many grams are covered by one unit (**A**):   **B / A** = a bolus of: _____ units of Humalog needed for this amount of carbohydrate

Take Bolus	Take your bolus and eat as planned

Check Blood Sugars

0 hour = _____ mg/dl (starting blood sugar)

1 hour = _____ mg/dl

2 hours = _____ mg/dl

3 hours = _____ mg/dl

3.5 hours = _____ mg/dl (ending blood sugar)

Check more often if your blood sugar is dropping quickly or may go low.

Stop the test if your blood sugar goes over 240 mg/dl (15 mmol) or below 65 mg/dl (3.6 mmol).

Analyze

After 3.5 hours, are you within 30 points (1.7 mmol) of your target?

▶   ▼   ◀

No, I'm more than 30 pts. below my target

Yes

No, I'm more than 30 pts. above my target

Retest again using a larger carb number--ie, if it was 1H/12 grams, use 1H/13 grams.

You have the correct insulin-to-carb ratio. Test two more times at different mealtimes to verify.

Retest again using a smaller carb number--ie, if it was 1H/12 grams, use 1H/11 grams.

is needed. If you choose not to adhere to the standard meal plan, and most people do not, do not continue taking set meal boluses.

Intentionally Reducing Boluses

When first starting on a pump, you may want to discount or reduce carb boluses. In other words, you might choose not to cover the first 10 grams of carbohydrate in your meals until you see how accurate your insulin-to-carb ratio is.

Bedtime boluses for snacks or high readings often are discounted to prevent night-time lows. This also can help balance increased activity or exercise that day. An easy way to reduce the bedtime dose is to cut it in half. For the sample pumper, 30 grams divided by 10 would be 3.0 units, but this is cut in half to 1.5 units at bedtime. Use this method, or discount by not covering the first 10 (or 20) grams as mentioned earlier.

Example of discounting for a person whose insulin-to carb ratio is 1 to 10:				
	Breakfast	Lunch	Dinner	Bedtime Snack
Carb Amount	40	60	60	30
Normal Bolus	40 / 10 = 4	60 / 10 = 6	60 / 10 = 6	30 / 10 = 3
Carbs less 10	30	50	50	20
Reduced Bolus	30 / 10 = 3	50 / 10 = 5	50 / 10 = 5	20 / 10 = 2

Timing Carb Boluses

Although the correct carb ratio is critical to good blood sugar control, another important factor is the timing of the bolus. Humalog's great advantage is the convenience of bolusing as you eat. Although Humalog can be given right before a meal, it prevents post meal highs best when it is bolused 15 to 30 minutes before eating. Humalog's action time parallels the digestion and absorption of most meals.

Regular insulin works best when it is bolused 30 to 45 minutes before eating. When Regular is not bolused early enough, the blood sugar may spike to high levels one to two hours after eating.

If your blood sugar is high before a meal and your schedule allows, take your meal bolus early enough, depending on how high the blood sugar is, to lower it before you begin eating. Post-meal readings can be improved if you can bring your blood sugar below 150 mg/dl (8.3 mmol) before eating. Set an alarm, so you do not delay your eating any longer than planned, since this can trigger a severe insulin reaction.

Whether using Humalog or Regular, if you are not sure when a meal will begin or what its carb content will be, you may not want to give the full carb bolus until you see the food on your plate. Being able to do this easily is one of the great advantages of using a pump. In this situation, you might give a partial bolus, perhaps half of the total amount that's anticipated for the meal. Then bolus the remainder when eating actually begins and the carbohydrate count is more certain. This allows the blood insulin level to rise by the time eating starts but reduces the risk of a low blood sugar. Fast-acting carbohydrates should always be available in case your blood sugar drops before the meal is actually served.

Remember that slight variations in your insulin-to-carb ratio may occur for food eaten at different times during the day. Also, foods with the same amount of carbohydrate but different glycemic indexes may require different boluses. For instance, 50 grams of carbohydrate from kidney beans is unlikely to require as much insulin as 50 grams from pizza.

Extended, Square Wave, and Combination Boluses

Today's pumps have the ability to deliver boluses in a variety of ways. In most situations, boluses are best delivered as a normal bolus over a short period of time. The advantage of this approach is that most meals are digested and enter the bloodstream faster than a Humalog bolus can be absorbed. Most carbohydrate-based foods are digested and turned into glucose within an hour and a half to three hours of eating. Even fast-acting Humalog cannot match these typical digestion times, so slowing bolus delivery would not make sense for most meals.

At times, however, food may be better matched by boluses that are extended or given over a longer period of time. Examples may include brunches where food is eaten in smaller amounts over several hours, very low glycemic index foods like red lentils that raise the blood sugar for several hours, and high protein foods like steak that convert to glucose over several hours following consumption. Individual pumpers will find that certain meals may be better covered with a temporary basal rate or an extended bolus due to these delayed blood sugar effects. Some pumps have a square wave or extended bolus feature which handles this situation nicely.

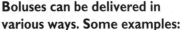

Boluses can be delivered in various ways. Some examples:

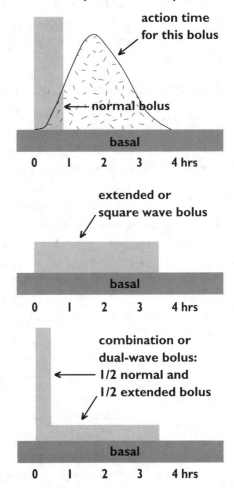

The rectangular shapes picture delivery of boluses, not their absorption which extends some 3.5 hours with Humalog.

Gastroparesis, a condition in which damage has occurred to the nerves that control digestion, is another situation where an extended bolus can be helpful. Unfortunately, gastroparesis is often unpredictable. Some pumpers with gastroparesis find that an extended bolus or temporary basal increase covers their delayed digestion very well. Others find that their digestion is so unpredictable that meals may be better covered by giving a combination bolus which is a reduced bolus, followed by either a corrective bolus or a smaller extended bolus after the blood sugar is checked two hours after the meal. Discuss these options with your physician/health care team and experiment to see which works best.

Convenience can be an asset but also a liability with a pump. Meal boluses may be forgotten, especially by harried parents, busy professionals, older pumpers, and teens. If you are a parent, you can expect that your child will forget to bolus occasionally. Luckily, the memory in today's pumps provides a convenient way to confirm recent boluses. The amount and timing of the last dozen or more boluses can be reviewed to see if a bolus was given. This memory provides a useful tool for parents and clinicians to verify whether boluses have been taken.

Test Your Insulin-To-Carb Ratio With Continuous Monitoring

Today's continuous monitors can easily test your insulin-to-carb ratio because you can see immediately the effect that carbs have on your blood sugars when readings are given several times an hour. Deciding how to react effectively to this much data is important. Frequent monitoring allows you to see the full impact of a bolus, but it is important to wait to let its full impact be seen. For instance, with Humalog, 3.5 hours is a good time to wait to see the full interaction of a meal and bolus. The ability to test this often allows you to wait, unless a low blood sugar occurs or a reading goes above 240 mg/dl (15 mmol) to 300 mg/dl (16.7 mmol).

The value of so many readings is that you can adjust your insulin-to-carb ratio specifically to the meal you are eating, especially if this information is recorded. You can identify foods that have a low glycemic index for you and match them differently than ones with a high glycemic index.

In fact, you can run your own experiment and see if the glucose from a specific food enters your own bloodstream in a fashion similar to its ranking in the glycemic index in this book. When your insulin-to-carb ratio is correct, a bolus will take your blood sugar from a starting value of say 100 mg/dl to 100 mg/dl 3.5 hours later, while the area under the curve between these two values reveals the food's glycemic index.

Meals that are a mixture of carbs, fats, protein, and fiber can also be matched. Continuous monitoring will enable you to specifically tailor your boluses to different meals with an extended bolus or combination bolus, as needed, so that the meal has a limited impact on your blood sugar. Continuous monitoring allows you to identify other food effects, such as the insulin-blocking action of certain fatty foods, that often causes the blood sugar to rise for several hours following foods like chips or meat pizza.

112

Tips On Carb Boluses

- Test how many carbs are covered by each unit of Humalog or Regular only after you have correctly set and tested your basal rates.

- Count carbs in each meal or snack. Estimate your carb boluses using the 500 Rule.

- The correct insulin-to-carb ratio for Humalog returns the blood sugar to within 30 points of the original blood sugar 3.5 hours after eating. (5 hrs. for Regular)

- Premeal boluses are determined before meals by the carbohydrate contained in the meal, with adjustments made for the current blood sugar reading and any planned activity.

- Signs of an incorrect insulin-to-carb ratio:

    Too little Humalog or Regular: the blood sugar is OK before meals or snacks but goes high after meals and does not drop before the next meal (or at bedtime).

    Too much Humalog or Regular: the blood sugar is OK before meals or snacks but drops too much one to four hours after food is eaten.

- Higher basal rates and extended boluses, or square wave boluses are useful for handling eating events that cover several hours, such as snacking, parties, or progressive dinners.

- Discount bolus coverage when first starting on a pump and when necessary as a short-term way to prevent lows. Discount bedtime boluses for safety.

Quick Basal Check:

Do your carb boluses make up 40% to 55% of your TDD?

Always plan ahead, it wasn't raining when Noah built the ark.

Richard Cushing

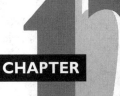

CHAPTER

Setting And Testing
High Blood Sugar Boluses

Besides carb coverage, boluses from a pump serve another important function. They are used to bring down high blood sugars quickly and safely. If you know how far your blood sugar drops on each unit of bolused insulin, you can bring any high blood sugar down to normal. After setting your basals and carb boluses, this is the last piece of your control puzzle: knowing how far your blood sugar drops for each unit of insulin.

This chapter shows:

- How to determine how far your blood sugar drops on each unit of insulin
- How much high blood sugar bolus to add to a carb bolus for a premeal high
- How much high blood sugar bolus to take for a high after a meal
- How to test your high blood sugar boluses

Set your blood sugar goals with help from your physician/health care team, who will tailor them to your special needs. For example, during pregnancy, a woman requires lower target blood sugars, while someone who has a history of hypoglycemia unawareness will want higher targets. After first starting on a pump, be extra cautious when taking a high blood sugar bolus. Test your blood sugar every hour for 3 to 4 hours after taking a Humalog bolus (every hour for 5 hours with Regular) to pick up the trend in your readings and avoid lows or continuing highs. Use Workspace 12.3 on page 122 to pick up trends in your dropping blood sugar. If the blood sugar is high at bedtime, a good rule of thumb for preventing nighttime lows is to take half of your usual high blood sugar bolus.

Continuous monitoring is a great aid in preventing high blood sugars, with an easy to see trend in your readings and an alarm feature to warn when your blood sugar rises above a selected upper limit. If you do have a high blood sugar, take a corrective bolus and track its effect as you avoid causing a low. The low alarm can also warn you if it drops below a selected lower limit.

Lower Highs With The 1500 And 1800 Rules

The 1500 Rule was the first tool that allowed precise dosing for high blood sugars. It was developed in the early 1990s by Paul C. Davidson, M.D., Medical Director of the Diabetes Treatment Center at HCA West Paces Ferry Hospital in Atlanta.[67] He based his "1500 Rule" on his experience with people with diabetes. When 1500 is divided by a person's total daily dose of insulin, the resulting number gives how far a blood sugar reading will be lowered by 1 unit of Regular insulin.

Use The 1800 Rule To Estimate Your Point Drop

To estimate your point drop per unit of Humalog, divide 1800 by your TDD (divide 1500 by TDD if on Regular)

Example:

If someone's TDD = 30 units

1800/30 = a 60 point drop per unit of Humalog

or 1500/30 = 50 point drop per unit of Regular

When your point drop per unit is known, an accurate high blood sugar scale can be set up to lower highs safely!

If you use faster-acting Humalog insulin, the number 1800 works better. With Humalog's faster onset and shorter action time, less Humalog than Regular is generally needed to lower high blood sugars. The number 1800 is used to estimate the point drop in Table 10.1. Based on your TDD, Table 12.1 gives suggested point drops for both Humalog and Regular insulin.

For instance, if a 160 pound person uses 40 units of Humalog as his/her TDD with 60% as basal, 40 units a day would be divided into 1800 to give a point drop of 45 mg/dl (2.5 mmol) per unit of Humalog. If a blood sugar before a meal were 280 mg/dl (15.6 mmol) and his/her target blood sugar were 100 mg/dl (5.6 mmol), an 180 point drop (10 mmol) would be desired. 180 points divided by 45 points per unit equals 4 units, so 4 units of Humalog would be added to the premeal bolus to correct the high.

What If I Measure BG In Millimoles?

For those who use millimoles, instead of the 1500 and 1800 Rules, the 84 Rule works well for Regular and the 100 Rule for Humalog. For instance, if your TDD is 25 units of Humalog per day in your pump, your blood sugar will drop 4 mmol (100/25 u/day = 4 mmol) on each unit of Humalog.

In this situation when the blood sugar is 280 (15.6 mmol), an individual's high blood sugar ratio can be tested by taking 4 units to bring down the high, eating no food and taking no carb bolus. If the blood sugar falls in three and a half hours to 100 mg/dl (5.6 mmol), this pumper knows his/her high blood sugar actually drops 45 mg/dl (2.5 mmol) for each unit of Humalog. A safe and appropriate high blood sugar scale can then be set up.

The number of points your own blood sugar will drop per unit depends largely on your TDD. For instance, someone using only 30 units of total insulin per day is likely to be thin and sensitive to insulin. This person's blood sugar will drop farther on one unit of Humalog, usually around 60 points (4.2 mmol) using the 1800 Rule, than someone who is insulin resistant and needs 100 units of insulin per day. The second person will have a blood sugar drop of about 18 points (1 mmol) per unit of

Table 12.1 Estimate Your Point Drop Per Unit Of Humalog Or Regular With 1800 Or 1500 Rule		
	1800 Rule	**1500 Rule**
For this TDD:	**On Humalog, Your Point Drop is:**	**On Regular, Your Point Drop is:**
16 units	1 H/112 pt. drop	1 H/94 pt. drop
18 units	1 H/100 pt. drop	1 H/83 pt. drop
20 units	1 H/90 pt. drop	1 H/75 pt. drop
22 units	1 H/82 pt. drop	1 H/68 pt. drop
24 units	1 H/75 pt. drop	1 H/63 pt. drop
26 units	1 H/69 pt. drop	1 H/58pt. drop
28 units	1 H/64 pt. drop	1 H/54 pt. drop
30 units	1 H/60 pt. drop	1 H/50 pt. drop
32 units	1 H/56 pt. drop	1 H/47 pt. drop
36 units	1 H/50 pt. drop	1 H/42 pt. drop
40 units	1 H/45 pt. drop	1 H/38 pt. drop
44 units	1 H/41 pt. drop	1 H/34 pt. drop
48 units	1 H/38 pt. drop	1 H/31 pt. drop
52 units	1 H/35 pt. drop	1 H/29 pt. drop
56 units	1 H/32 pt. drop	1 H/27 pt. drop
60 units	1 H/30 pt. drop	1 H/25 pt. drop
65 units	1 H/28 pt. drop	1 H/23 pt. drop
70 units	1 H/26 pt. drop	1 H/21 pt. drop
75 units	1 H/24 pt. drop	1 H/20 pt. drop
80 units	1 H/22 pt. drop	1 H/19 pt. drop
90 units	1 H/20 pt. drop	1 H/17 pt. drop
100 units	1 H/18 pt. drop	1 H/15 pt. drop

Humalog and will need a bolus that is at least 3 times as large as that used by the first individual to lower the same high blood sugar.

The 1800 and 1500 Rules for determining the point drop per unit of Humalog or Regular may not be as accurate for Type 2s as for Type 1s because of the extra internal insulin production that is not taken into account. However, at the worst, these Rules will underestimate insulin need, so that insulin reactions are unlikely.

How To Test High Blood Sugar Boluses

After you estimate how far your blood sugars fall per unit of insulin from Table 10.1, test this estimate to see whether it is accurate. Set up your sliding scale with your physician's help, selecting appropriate pre-meal and post-meal targets. Then test it as described below and adjust as needed.

Workspace 12.1 on page 119 shows how to test high blood sugar boluses. With your physician's help, select your ideal target blood sugar before meals. This target is usually between 90 mg/dl (5 mmol) and 140 mg/dl (7.8 mmol) for testing purposes. If you use Humalog, the test can be started whenever a premeal blood sugar is above 200 mg/dl (11.1 mmol) provided it has been at least three and a half hours since the last Humalog bolus was given, and at least two hours since the last food was eaten. Once you start the test, delay eating for three and a half hours until testing is completed or your blood sugar goes low.

If you use Regular, the test can be conducted when a blood sugar is above 200 mg/dl (11.1 mmol), but at least five hours must have passed since the last Regular bolus was given and two hours since the last food was eaten. Eating has to be delayed for another five hours to complete the test with Regular.

> **Remember:** Always set and test your basal rates before attempting to determine your carb boluses or high blood sugar boluses. The amount of Humalog or Regular needed for meals and high blood sugars can be determined only after the basal insulin has been set correctly.

This test is repeated until a ratio is found that brings your blood sugar to within 30 mg/dl of your target on two consecutive tests started 3.5 hours after the Humalog bolus is taken and without triggering an insulin reaction. Test the blood sugar often during the test to catch and treat any low blood sugar that might occur. On Regular, the test is successful if the blood sugar is within 30 points after 5 hours.

Once your point drop has been determined through testing, you can create your own personalized high blood sugar scale. This scale is one of the most important tools for helping you fine tune your blood sugar control. The ability to lower high blood sugars safely is the last major skill needed for excellent control.

To set up your scale, first select with your physician your ideal or target blood sugars for before meals and after meals. Since your blood sugar naturally rises after

Workspace 12.1 How To Test Your Point Drop Per Unit On Humalog

Prepare

With your doctor, decide on a target blood sugar level before meals (usually 90 to 140 mg/dl, or 5 to 7.8 mmol):

_____ mg/dl = my target

Use Table 10.1 or Table 12.1 and your physician's help to decide how many points your blood sugar is likely to drop per unit of Humalog.

_____ mg/dl = my point drop/unit of H (**A**)

Be sure 3.5 hours have passed since your last bolus and 3 hours since eating food.

Start

When your blood sugar is above 200 mg/dl (11.1 mmol) and you can wait 3.5 hours to eat.

Do The Math

1. From your current high reading, subtract your target blood sugar:

My current blood sugar: _____ mg/dl

minus my target blood sugar: _____ mg/dl

equals: _____ points to drop (**B**)

2. Divide the points you want to drop (**B**) by how many points your blood sugar is likely to drop per unit (**A**):

B / A = a bolus of: _____ units of Humalog needed to lower your blood sugar to your target

Take Bolus

Take this bolus to correct high blood sugar, unless it seems to be wrong!

Check Blood Sugars

1 hour = _____ mg/dl

2 hours = _____ mg/dl

3 hours = _____ mg/dl

3.5 hours = _____ mg/dl

Check more often if your blood sugar is dropping quickly or may go low.

Stop the test if your blood sugar does not come down or is low.

Analyze

After 3.5 hours, are you within 30 points (1.7 mmol) of your target?

▶ ▼ ◀

No, I'm more than 30 pts. below my target

Retest another time using a larger point drop number-ie, if it was 1H/40 pts, use 1H/43 pts

Yes

You have the correct ratio for your point drop per unit of H. Test again to verify, then use it to set up your personal high blood sugar bolus scale in Workspace 12.2.

No, I'm more than 30 pts. above my target

Retest another time using a smaller point drop number-ie, if it was 1H/40 pts, use 1H/37 pts eating, your target following a meal will be higher than your before-meal target. For instance, a target of 100 mg/dl (5.6 mmol) before eating and 150 mg/dl (10 mmol) two hours after eating is reasonable for many pumpers using Humalog.

It is important to realize that if the bolus insulin that you actually need to lower your blood sugars differs significantly from the

Workspace 12.2 A Scale To Lower High Blood Sugars

Use the value found with your testing in Workspace 12.1 to set up a personal high blood sugar bolus scale. The points you drop per unit should remain the same for before and after meal readings, but your target blood sugar will change. For example, your target might be 100 mg/dl (5.6 mmol) before meals and 180 mg/dl (10 mmol) after.

My blood sugar goals

Premeal: 1 H for each _____ mg/dl   over _____ mg/dl **before** meals

or over _____ mg/dl **after** meals

If my blood sugar is:	I will correct by giving this extra bolus:	
	before meals	**at bedtime or 2 hrs. after meals**
100 mg/dl	no extra	no extra
_____ mg/dl	_____ extra units	no extra
_____ mg/dl	_____ extra units	no extra
_____ mg/dl	_____ extra units	_____ extra units
_____ mg/dl	_____ extra units	_____ extra units
_____ mg/dl	_____ extra units	_____ extra units
_____ mg/dl	_____ extra units	_____ extra units
_____ mg/dl	_____ extra units	_____ extra units
_____ mg/dl	_____ extra units	_____ extra units
_____ mg/dl	_____ extra units	_____ extra units

amount predicted in Table 10.1 (pg. 92), it is likely that your TDD is incorrect, or your basal rate may need to be retested.

If your blood sugar is unacceptably high but you have recently taken another bolus for any reason, you must take this still-active insulin into account when determining this particular high blood sugar bolus. You do this by applying the unused bolus rule that is described in the next chapter.

A Sample High Blood Sugar Scale

Your own high blood sugar scale for pre-meals and post-meals can be set up, using the information in Table 12.1 on page 117, once you have tested the recommended number and found it to be accurate. Remember that the size of the Humalog bolus you need to bring a high blood sugar down to normal is determined by how far above a selected target your blood sugar is, by how many points your blood sugar will drop on each unit of Humalog, and by whether this is a pre- or post-meal high.

Table 12.2 shows a sample high blood sugar bolus scale. This particular person weighs 160 pounds and has good control, using 40 units of insulin a day with 60% of the TDD as basal. The scale was created by referring to Table 10.1 or Table 12.1 to determine that this person's blood sugar was likely to drop about 45 points for each unit of Humalog. The target blood sugars were chosen with his physician's help: 100 mg/dl (5.6 mmol) before meals and 180 mg/dl (10 mmol) two hours after meals. This sample scale gives the dose of Humalog, in half unit increments, that will be needed for high blood sugars that might occur either before or after meals.

Table 12.2 Sample High BG Scale		
If Blood Sugar (mg/dl) is:	Additional Bolus Needed	
	Before Meal	After Meal
100-119	0	0
120-139	0.5 unit	0
140-159	1.0 unit	0
160-179	1.5 units	0
180-199	2.0 units	0.5 unit
200-219	2.5 units	1.0 unit
220-239	3.0 units	1.5 units
240-259	3.5 units	2.0 units
260-279	4.0 units	2.5 units
280-299	4.5 units	3.0 units
300-319	5.0 units	3.5 units
320-339	5.5 units	4.0 units
340-359	6.0 units	4.5 units

A good clue that your TDD is correctly set is that you rarely need to use a high blood sugar bolus and rarely need treatment for low blood sugars.

Do not use the 1500 or 1800 Rule to lower high blood sugars:

- before discussing it with your physician.
- if your high blood sugars tend to come down on their own.
- if you have frequent or severe lows.

For premeal highs, the extra high blood sugar bolus can be added to the carb bolus given for the meal. You would not use an extra Humalog for a high blood sugar, of course, if your blood sugars fall from high readings to normal on their own, which suggests that your basal rates are too high. Another situation in which you would not need as much extra insulin is if you planned to exercise soon after the meal.

Only experience can tell you when you need a bolus for a high blood sugar that occurs between meals. In some situations, as when a meal bolus was forgotten and taken just after eating, a blood sugar of 200 or 300 mg/dl (11.1 to 16.7 mmol) at one or two hours after the meal might be ignored because the blood sugar will return to normal as the late bolus begins to take effect.

In many circumstances, however, blood sugars of 200 or 300 mg/dl following a meal will not return to normal unless a high blood sugar bolus is taken. It is important to understand what your own blood sugars do, and to have an individualized high blood sugar bolus table to guide you in taking the correct bolus. As with all insulin doses, be sure to get personal guidance from your physician/health care team.

Workspace 12.3 Plot Your High BG Bolus Test Results

After taking a bolus to lower a high blood sugar, test every 30 to 60 min. Connect your readings with a line to see your trend.

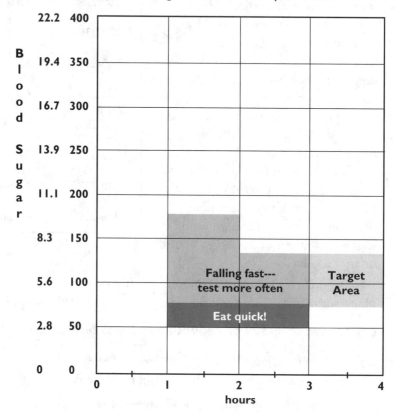

As you test your high blood sugar bolus using Workspace 12.1, check your sugar at least every hour. Plot your results on this graph and check that the line between your readings is heading toward the target area. If not, begin testing more often.

Caution

One post-meal blood sugar situation you will encounter sooner or later deserves special caution. Suppose you forget your carb bolus before a meal entirely

and when you check your blood sugar two hours later, you find it very high. How much bolus insulin should you take? Many pumpers think they should take their forgotten carb bolus along with a high blood sugar bolus to bring the blood sugar down. **Do not do this!**

The blood sugar is high because the carb bolus was forgotten, but these carbs are already digested and are obviously already in your blood causing the blood sugar to be high The only insulin needed in this situation is a high blood sugar bolus to bring your blood sugar down. Do not take any bolus to cover the already digested carbohydrates. Instead, in this situation use your premeal high blood sugar scale because there has been no recent carb bolus to help lower your post-meal high blood sugar. The smaller post-meal type of bolus won't be able to do the job alone.

How far the blood sugar drops on a unit of Humalog or Regular generally stays the same, unless infection, ketoacidosis, a marked change in physical activity, or other complicating factors are present. If your blood sugar drop per unit of Humalog or Regular varies greatly from one time of day to another, you may want to retest your basal rates to make sure they have been set accurately.

What To Do About Frequent High Blood Sugars

High blood sugar boluses are intended to correct occasional high blood sugars, but sometimes pumpers find they need to use corrective boluses every day. This is a very good indication that the TDD is too low. An increased need for insulin may be caused by growth in children and adolescents, weight gain, reduced activity, increased stress, or seasonal changes. Whatever the reason, when high blood sugar boluses are required frequently, this strongly suggests that your TDD needs to be increased. Chapter 14 gives some guidelines for when and how much your TDD should be changed.

When frequent corrections are needed, look to see whether there is any pattern to them. For instance, if highs seem to occur at almost all times of day, increase your TDD evenly between the basals and boluses. If your highs are almost always before breakfast, the nighttime basal rate is likely to need raising, while if your dinner readings are usually the culprit, try raising the afternoon basal and the lunch bolus.

Be careful in raising your TDD. For instance, if you need high blood sugar boluses every day simply to lower highs that are caused because you are overtreating frequent lows, an insulin reduction may be more appropriate.

Tips On High Blood Sugar Boluses

• The correct ratio of Humalog or Regular to the number of points (mg/dl or mmol) the blood sugar drops will bring a high blood sugar to within 30 points of the target blood sugar three and a half hours with Humalog and five hours with Regular.

• The point drop per unit of insulin is generally stable and predictable. However, certain situations like ketoacidosis, infections, increased weight, or less activity will reduce the number of points the blood sugar will drop per unit. On the other hand, a loss of weight or increase in activity will lower your TDD, and this will increase the fall in blood sugar per unit. Frequent testing can be very helpful.

• If an unexpected high blood sugar occurs, always try to determine the cause. It may be interrupted insulin delivery or bad insulin that is causing the problem.

• Signs that your high blood sugar bolus ratio may be incorrect:

Your high blood sugars often do not drop to your target suggesting your bolus contains too little insulin.

Your high blood sugar often drops below your target or drops sooner than expected, suggesting your bolus contains too much insulin.

• Boluses used to lower high blood sugars are not included as part of your TDD. Any time you find you need frequent high blood sugar boluses, suspect that your TDD is too low. Recalculate your TDD and raise both your basals and boluses appropriately.

• Be cautious when correcting high blood sugars at or near bedtime to reduce your risk of a nighttime insulin reaction. Use the unused bolus rule in the next chapter to determine how much bolus insulin given earlier in the evening may still be active at bedtime.

Live more from imagination than from memory.

Stephen Covey

The Unused Bolus Rule

A great advantage of pump therapy is that boluses can be given easily at any time a need arises. A bolus for dinner, another for an unplanned dessert, another for the high blood sugar that follows. However, when boluses begin to overlap, a problem surfaces. How much insulin is still working from recent boluses? You need to know this to prevent giving too much insulin and to avoid unnecessary low blood sugars.

Determining residual insulin is always important, but especially at bedtime. If several boluses have been given over the evening hours, the bedtime blood sugar has to be interpreted in light of how much insulin is still working. A normal blood sugar at bedtime may be dangerous if you still have a large residual bolus working. Likewise, a high reading at bedtime may require no additional bolus if the residual bolus will be taking care of it.

This chapter explains:

- The unused bolus rule
- How to determine how much insulin or carbohydrate is needed in situations where recent boluses are still active
- How to apply the unused bolus tables

What Is The Unused Bolus Rule?

The unused bolus rule lets you estimate how many units of Humalog or Regular insulin are still working from your recent boluses. Most people find that a bolus of Humalog starts working 15 minutes after the bolus is given, peaks in activity at one and a half hours, and is gone after three and a half hours. A bolus of Regular starts working a half hour after the injection, peaks two to three hours later, and stops dropping the blood sugar after five to six hours. From these action times we get the unused bolus rule:

> For Humalog, 30% of a bolus is used each hour after the bolus.
>
> For Regular, 20% of a bolus is used each hour after the bolus.

These rules help in determining how much residual insulin is still working at any time after a bolus. With Humalog, approximately 30% of a bolus is used each hour, and with Regular, about 20% is used per hour.

In some individuals, Regular insulin may work longer than five hours. If you are older or take larger doses, you may find a bolus of Regular is still lowering the blood sugar even six or seven hours after it was given. If this is the case, you may want to estimate an unused bolus rule that uses 16 percent or one sixth of the Regular bolus per hour as your guide. Alternatively, you may decide to simply switch to Humalog, which tends to work consistently over three and a half to four hours no matter how large the bolus.

Table 13.1 Insulin Activity At 1, 2, 3, and 4 Hours After A Bolus With Humalog				
Original Bolus Amount	Units Of Humalog Left After:			
	1 Hr	2 Hrs	3 Hrs	4 Hrs
1 unit	0.7	0.4	0.1	0
2 units	1.4	0.8	0.2	0
3 units	2.1	1.2	0.3	0
4 units	2.8	1.6	0.4	0
5 units	3.5	2.0	0.5	0
6 units	4.2	2.4	0.6	0
7 units	4.9	2.8	0.7	0
8 units	5.6	3.2	0.8	0
9 units	6.3	3.6	0.9	0
10 units	7.0	4.0	1.0	0

How To Find Unused Boluses

Tables 13.1 for Humalog and 13.2 for Regular provide a convenient interpretation of the unused bolus rule. Be sure to discuss use of these tables with your physician.

With the unused bolus rule and knowing how far your blood sugar drops on each unit of Humalog, you are able to determine

- how much insulin is still working from recent boluses
- how much additional bolus may be needed to lower a high blood sugar
- whether carbohydrate may be needed to avoid a low because too much insulin may have been given

Example One: Let's say your blood sugar is off your meter's scale, somewhere above 450 mg/dl or 25 mmol (ketones negative, pump working). Since your blood sugar drops 40 points per unit (a TDD of 45 units), you take 9 units of Humalog to bring the high reading down. You check your blood sugar again in two hours and find it now measures 344 mg/dl (19.1 mmol). Do you need to take another Humalog bolus?

To find out, let's use Table 13.1 for Humalog. Using this table, you find that after two hours, 60 percent of your previous Humalog bolus is gone. You took 9 units, so 9 units X .60 = 5.4 units have been used. That means that 9 units minus 5.4 units or 3.6 units of Humalog are left to work. (See Table 13.1 for confirmation.)

Since your blood sugar drops 40 points (2.2 mmol) on each unit of Humalog, you now can calculate the activity left from your 9 unit bolus:

Original Bolus Amount	Units Of Regular Left After:				
	1 Hr	2 Hrs	3 Hrs	4 Hrs	5 Hrs
1 unit	0.8	0.6	0.4	0.2	0
2 units	1.6	1.2	0.8	0.4	0
3 units	2.4	1.8	1.2	0.6	0
4 units	3.2	2.4	1.6	0.8	0
5 units	4.0	3.0	2.0	1.0	0
6 units	4.8	3.6	2.4	1.2	0
7 units	5.6	4.2	2.8	1.4	0
8 units	6.4	4.8	3.2	1.6	0
9 units	7.2	5.4	3.6	1.8	0
10 units	8.0	6.0	4.0	2.0	0

Table 13.2 Insulin Activity At 1, 2, 3, 4, and 5 Hours After A Bolus With Regular

3.6 units left times 40 points dropped per unit equals 144 points (8 mmol)

Your blood sugar is likely to drop another 144 points because of your bolus. Since your blood sugar is 344 (19.1 mmol), you can expect to be at 344 – 144, or 200 mg/dl (11.1 mmol) in a little over an hour when the last of the 9 unit bolus of Humalog is used up. Knowing this, you know you're likely to need an additional bolus to finish correcting this high blood sugar. You then can calculate the second Humalog bolus needed to lower your blood sugar as follows:

200 minus 100 (your target blood sugar) equals 100 more points you want to drop

100 points ÷ 40 points per unit = 2.5 more units to bring the blood sugar down.

These calculations depend on having your basal and bolus doses correctly set (i.e., your blood sugars are generally well controlled), and no other problems such as a loose hub, leaky O-rings, or bad insulin. When taking any boluses using the unused bolus rule, test your blood sugar more frequently. To avoid nighttime insulin reactions, reduce boluses for highs at bedtime, taking perhaps half of what you would take normally, and set your alarm to wake you in 2 or 3 hours to check for a low blood sugar. At this time use the unused bolus rule again to determine if any additional drop is likely.

Example Two: As another example, let's say you go out for breakfast at a new restaurant. After ordering pancakes and fruit, you delay your bolus until your food arrives to be sure how many carbohydrates it will have. When your plate arrives, you estimate 100 grams and take a 9 unit bolus of Humalog (i.e., your TDD is 45 units with 1 H for each 11 grams). However, two hours later when you measure your blood sugar, you find it is 200 mg/dl (11.1 mmol). You know that your blood sugar drops 40 points on each unit of Humalog. Do you need to do anything with this blood sugar?

To find out, let's first determine how much insulin is left from the breakfast bolus using the unused bolus rule. You took 9 units an hour and a half ago, so roughly 60 percent (30 percent times 2 hours) has been used. This leaves 40 percent of the meal bolus still left to work. From Table 13.2:

9 units times 0.4 equals 3.6 units still active

As this bolus continues to work over the next two hours, your blood sugar should drop an additional 144 points (40 point drop per unit times 3.6 units left). Therefore, when the bolus is totally gone, your blood sugar should be

200 minus the final 144 points or 56 (predicted blood sugar).

This tells us the elevated blood sugar would come down on its own. A followup blood sugar in 60 minutes will clarify whether this is happening. You may see that you will need a small amount of carbohydrate to avoid a mild low blood sugar.

This example indicates why you should think twice about using a high blood sugar bolus. It takes at least two hours to get an idea of what the last carb or high blood sugar bolus is doing if you are using Humalog, and three hours if it is Regular. Taking boluses too soon after the meal can create an excess accumulation of insulin, complicate your bolus calculations, and create situations where insulin reactions become likely.

This example also illustrates a problem that often arises when eating out. In this situation, the post-meal blood sugar rises higher than a desirable target of 140 or 150 mg/dl (7.8 to 8.3 mmol) at two hours. This carb-rich breakfast could not be covered well even with what appears to be an adequate or slightly excessive bolus of Humalog because it was taken just before beginning to eat. In many situations like going out for a pancake breakfast, it helps to lead the meal with a partial bolus taken a half hour early. Of course, keep glucose tablets handy as needed.

14

When To Change Your TDD

Any time you experience control problems, check first to determine whether you are on the correct TDD. Your TDD from Workspace 9.1 (pg. 85) may have worked well at one time, but if changes have occurred in your life, your TDD will need to be changed also.

The most reliable sign that your insulin doses need to be changed is blood sugars that are frequently high or low. Frequent highs or lows can be caused by many things, but a consistent pattern of them tells you your TDD needs to be raised or lowered. For instance, frequent or severe lows almost always indicate that your TDD needs to be lowered. Determine what your current TDD is, reduce this amount by 10% using Table 14.1, then go back to Table 10.1 (pg. 92), and recalculate your basals and boluses using this new TDD. Frequent highs usually mean your TDD is too low and needs to be raised. Be sure to test your new basal rates and boluses before relying on them extensively.

When control problems occur, always think carefully about their cause. If you have been guessing the carbs in meals, your control may be improved simply by taking the time to count your carbs carefully and figuring appropriate boluses to cover them. Anytime you are having a pattern of highs or lows, such as when you need to take high blood sugar boluses more than once a day, or you are gaining weight because you are needing to compensate for lows frequently, your cause is a TDD in need of adjustment.

Always try to determine whether highs or lows are your primary problem. For instance, if you are almost always high, your TDD likely needs to be raised (or you may have a bad bottle of insulin). However frequent highs could result also from overtreating frequent lows, or from eating excess carbs to avoid low blood sugars. Under these circumstances, raising your TDD would not solve the problem.

How To Adjust Your TDD When Using A Pump And Control Is Poor

If you are having control problems while on a pump, your current TDD (basals and carb boluses) can provide an excellent guide to make adjustments to get yourself out of a pattern of highs or lows.

1. To start, to divide your weight in pounds by 4 (or, if you weigh in kilograms, divide your kilogram weight by 1.8) to find out what your TDD would be if you had an average sensitivity to insulin for a person of your weight. Or use Table 9.1 on page 86.

2. Next, determine your current TDD by adding up your typical daily basals and carb boluses. Most pumps provide a record of your TDD for each of the last few days. These can be averaged to provide an accurate estimate of your current TDD. Ordinarily, any extra boluses used to lower high blood sugars are not counted when you are deciding whether to raise or lower your TDD, although the amount of high blood sugar boluses you use a day gives some guidance. For instance, if on your current basals and boluses you have a TDD of 20 units a day, but you are using an additional 20 units a day to lower high blood sugars, your current TDD will likely need a major increase.

3. Next, increase or decrease your TDD to correct your control problem. If you are having occasional lows, use Table 14.1 to reduce your TDD by 5% and recalculate your basals and boluses. For frequent or severe lows, reduce your TDD by 10%. Similarly, if you are having occasional highs, increase your TDD by 5% or increase by 10% if highs are frequent or severe. Table 14.1 provides an easy way to figure the increase or decrease of your TDD.

4. Then use your new TDD with Table 10.1 (pg. 92) to find your new average basal rate and bolus ratios. Discuss with your physician exactly how your basals and boluses can be changed for the best effect. Test the new basal rate as outlined in Chapter 10, and retest your bolus ratios as outlined in Chapters 11 and 12, if these have also changed.

For safety's sake, first use the smallest TDD that seems likely to control your blood sugar. Ask your physician/health care team for assistance in figuring these adjustments. Their experience and feedback can speed your path to better control.

Reasons To Adjust Your TDD

There are many situations that make it necessary for you to change your TDD and corresponding basals and boluses. Some situations require that insulin doses be increased gradually over time, such as during a child's growth spurts or during a pregnancy. Other situations, like an infection or the use of a steroid prescription, may

How To Adjust Your TDD

When control problems occur, use this table to increase your TDD to stop highs or to decrease your TDD to stop lows. For instance, a 5% decrease might be used for someone experiencing mild hypoglycemia, while a 10% increase might be needed in someone experiencing frequent blood sugars above 200 mg/dl (11.1 mmol) with rare lows.

See also Chapter 24 for information on how to spot blood sugar patterns and use precise adjustments to correct control problems.

Remember, almost all pumpers will need between 45% to 60% of their TDD delivered as basal insulin, with the remainder given as carb boluses. Check your own basal/TDD ratio to be sure it is correctly set.

Table 14.1 How To Change Your Total Daily Dose To Correct Highs Or Lows

With frequent lows, decrease your TDD			If your Current TDD is:	With frequent highs, increase your TDD		
25% less	10% less	5% less		5% more	10% more	25% more
12	14	15	16 units	17	18	20
14	16	17	18 units	19	20	22
15	18	19	20 units	21	22	25
16	20	21	22 units	23	24	28
18	22	23	24 units	25	26	30
20	23	25	26 units	27	28	32
21	25	27	28 units	29	31	35
22	27	28	30 units	32	33	38
24	29	30	32 units	34	35	40
27	32	34	36 units	38	40	45
30	36	38	40 units	42	44	50
33	40	42	44 units	46	48	55
36	43	46	48 units	50	53	60
39	47	49	52 units	55	57	65
42	50	53	56 units	59	62	70
45	54	57	60 units	63	66	75
49	58	62	65 units	68	72	81
52	63	66	70 units	74	77	88
56	68	71	75 units	79	82	94
60	72	76	80 units	84	88	100
68	81	86	90 units	94	99	112
75	90	95	100 units	105	110	125

require an immediate and large increase in TDD. Still other situations that affect your TDD may be less obvious. A few of the more common ones are discussed here.

1. When your activity level changes

Physical activity and physical fitness determine much of your sensitivity to insulin. A marathon runner, for example, may need only half as much insulin circulating in the blood as a person who doesn't exercise regularly. The runner's need is lower because of a marked increase in sensitivity to insulin due to physical training. Whenever there's a substantial increase in fitness, a reduction in TDD will be required.

For example, if you work as a moderately active flight attendant and are going to spend two weeks bicycling, plan on lowering your TDD. Plan on just the opposite if your activity level decreases. If you worked as a framer on a construction crew, but now work at a desk as a project cost estimator, less physical activity will increase your need for insulin unless you substitute increased exercise for the lost work activity.

2. When your weight changes

Your bathroom scale provides a great gauge for your TDD. When you weigh more, you need more insulin. If your weight drops, your TDD will need to be lowered.

The speed of the weight change mirrors how quickly your insulin needs change. If swimsuit season is suddenly upon you, or you decide at the last moment to attend your high school reunion, or out-of-town relatives call to tell you they'll be visiting next month, weight-panic often sets in. Where did those extra pounds come from and how can they be shed quickly? You may reduce eating immediately in an effort to bring about a quick image change.

This type of weight loss is not recommended, but if you are determined to lose weight in this manner, be aware that your TDD also will need a quick reduction. You may find you need to reduce your TDD by 10% to 30% if you suddenly restrict calorie intake. Basal rates will need to be lowered, and so will bolus sizes due to less carbohydrate intake combined with the resultant increased sensitivity to insulin.

How much weight is lost or gained also is important. A gradual change of 5 pounds or so may have little effect on the TDD, but if the weight change is 10 pounds or more, an adjustment in the TDD likely will be needed.

3. Change in weather, season, or altitude

With the warmer weather and longer days of spring, less insulin is often needed. Most people are more active in the summertime, and they have less fat in their diet as well. Also, the body uses more energy to cool itself in hot weather.

Just the opposite usually happens with the approach of winter. More insulin is needed by most people, but if you are outside during very cold weather and find yourself shivering, you are using more energy to stay warm. This actually means you may need less insulin. Similarly, at higher altitudes more energy is needed to breath and pump blood because the air becomes thinner. Until your body acclimates to the altitude, which usually takes a few days, less TDD or more carbohydrate may be required.

4. Around menstrual periods

Many women find their blood sugar rises in the days just before their menstrual period begins. If this increase is small, it may not require increasing the TDD, but for many women a substantial increase in both basal and bolus insulin during the few days prior to their period improves premenstrual symptoms and blood sugar control. The need for extra insulin quickly returns to normal on the first day of your period; at that time insulin doses should be adjusted back to their previous levels. Be sure to check the blood sugar often as you make substantial changes in your TDD, basal rates, and boluses. Many of today's pumps offer two, three, or four basal profiles, and one of these alternate profiles can be set up for the increased insulin need seen around menses.

5. During an illness

Illnesses, especially bacterial infections, place extra stress on the body. A higher TDD with both larger boluses and higher basal rates is often needed to counteract this physical stress. This is especially true for bacterial infections, like pneumonia, a strep throat, an impacted wisdom tooth, a bladder infection or a sinus infection. These are often accompanied by a fever and can cause the need for insulin to double or triple. After an antibiotic has been started, however, any temporary increase in basal rates or boluses will have to be reduced quickly to prevent insulin reactions.

Illnesses that last several weeks, like hepatitis and mononucleosis, often require an increase in the basal rate. Shorter viral illnesses, like a cold or flu, have a more varied and milder effect on blood sugars. Control during short-term viral illnesses usually is easier to achieve by using a higher carb ratio or more high blood sugar boluses as needed rather than raising the basal rate. During an illness, extra bolus insulin may be needed for meals even though your eating is reduced. You will want to do lots of extra blood sugar testing to determine how to take the extra insulin you may require.

Illnesses that cause vomiting or diarrhea may mean you can't eat, but they do not affect the need for basal insulin. Eliminate carb boluses if you cannot eat, of course, but continue to take your basal insulin. Correct highs as needed. Be sure to test your blood sugar more often or have someone else test it during any illness. If your blood sugar is high and has been for a while, test for ketones and be sure to drink lots of liquids.

6. During stress

Mild emotions and excitement can lower blood sugars, but stress often raises them. Many times stress isn't obvious until after it has caused a rise in the blood sugar. When this happens, use a bolus to bring down the high blood sugar.

If you anticipate only a short period of stress, such as a day of tension-filled business meetings, check your blood sugar often and take a bolus if it goes high. If you are going through a long stressful period, such as having a family member in the hospital, consider raising your TDD and basal rate to help your control and coping skills. When possible, maintain or increase your exercise regimen when you are stressed as this will lessen the impact that stress would have otherwise.

7. When using certain medications

Certain drugs greatly increase the need for insulin. Paramount among these are steroids like prednisone and cortisone. Whether taken orally for poison ivy, for allergic reactions to medications, and for illnesses such as lupus or asthma, or as an injection into an inflamed joint, steroids generally make insulin need rise sharply. One of us (the one with diabetes) got a severe case of poison oak while clearing fire brush out of a field, which required taking prednisone tablets for a few days. This caused a very substantial rise in blood sugars and insulin requirements. To control these high blood sugars, TDD and basal rates were raised and larger boluses were taken, some of which were 4 and 5 times those normally used.

Occasionally, the physician who prescribes oral or injected steroids for medical problems may be unaware how dramatically they can affect blood sugar levels. Steroids injected into joints will usually increase insulin need for 3 to 5 days. If steroids are required, make sure the physician prescribing them is aware of your diabetes to coordinate any increase in your insulin doses. Contact your diabetes physician/health care team as soon as possible to discuss the insulin adjustments that will be needed.

8. With thyroid disease

Thyroid disease occurs fairly often with both types of diabetes. It occurs with Type 2 because both thyroid disease and Type 2 are more common as we age. In fact, one out of every 10 women over age 65 has thyroid disease. It is more common in Type 1 because Type 1 and thyroid disease can both result from an autoimmune attack on hormone-producing glands.

Thyroid disease occurs gradually over a period of weeks or months. It may begin as a release of too much thyroid, then gradually change to too little. Because thyroid disease occurs gradually and may cause high (overactive thyroid) or low (underactive thyroid) blood sugars, the reason for the loss of control often is difficult to identify. If your blood sugars have changed and you have thyroid symptoms like nervousness, feeling hot or cold, tiredness or sleeping difficulties, have your thyroid checked.

If you have a low thyroid level and are placed on thyroid medication, you will probably need to raise your insulin doses slightly to control your blood sugars, especially if you have adjusted your insulin doses downward as your thyroid became less active. If you have an overactive thyroid and take radioactive iodine or undergo surgery to knock out part of the excess thyroid production, you may need to lower your basals and boluses. This is especially true if you have gradually increased your TDD as your thyroid production gradually increased.

9. With gastroparesis

Gastroparesis or paralysis of the intestines is damage to the nerves that control the wavelike motion of the intestines. This disorder delays the absorption of food after a meal. When a person with gastroparesis gives a bolus to cover a meal, they will often experience low blood sugars at 2 to 3 hours, followed by high blood sugars 6 or 8 hours later as the food is finally absorbed and converted to glucose in the blood.

This disorder does not change TDD as much as it may necessitate a slight reduction in TDD, or a redistribution of basals and boluses. A person with gastroparesis may benefit from a higher than normal daytime basal rate, perhaps as high as 70% of the TDD. The basal rate may be raised from early morning through the late evening to counter slowly digesting carbs, with meal boluses greatly reduced.

Today's pumps can also delay the delivery of boluses to match delayed absorption of food due either to gastroparesis or a low glycemic index. An extended or square wave bolus can be tailored with dosing and timing changes to almost any situation. See more information about alternate bolus delivery on pages 111 and 112.

Keep in mind that most blood sugar problems have nothing to do with gastroparesis, even though this condition is not rare. Symptoms that suggest the presence of gastroparesis include feeling full, a mild stomach pain, a feeling of fullness after eating, always feeling full, excess gas, bloating, nausea and vomiting.

Gastroparesis is almost always accompanied by other signs of damage to the autonomic nerves, such as loss of constriction of the pupils to light, loss of variability in the heart rate, and inability of the blood vessels to constrict when going from reclining in bed to standing. Signals indicating that autonomic neuropathy is present include light-headedness when first standing up, a heart rate that does not rise appropriately when exercising, sweating after eating, and impotence.

Fortunately, simple tests can determine whether gastroparesis is a cause of blood sugar control problems. On a standard EKG test, if the QTc interval, which measures how long it takes the heart muscle to lose its electrical charge after a heart beat, is longer than 0.44 seconds, autonomic neuropathy is suggested. Another test is the heart rate variability seen after deep breathing (Valsalva maneuver), or on a 24-hour Holter monitor during daily activities.

After lying down for a few minutes, a simple blood pressure check done while reclining can be compared to another done just after standing. If the difference in blood pressures shows more than a 20 point drop in the upper blood pressure number, or more than a 10 point drop in the lower blood pressure number, this suggests autonomic neuropathy. Consult your physician if you believe gastroparesis may be contributing to control problems.

Summary

Whenever your control is not what you desire, always consider starting from scratch. Determine your TDD, then set and test your basal rates, set and test your carb boluses, and finally figure your high blood sugar boluses. Reset and retest until your control is really improved. Consider different basal rates for different times of the 24-hour period. Make only one change at a time and see the effects for several days before moving on. Be patient and keep looking until you find an approach that helps your control, and most importantly, stay in close contact with your health care team.

Quit worrying about your health. It'll go away.

Fletcher Knebel

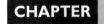

Insulin Reactions

Most people who use insulin are concerned about insulin reactions. Mild reactions can be annoying or embarrassing, while a severe reaction can be uncomfortable, frightening, and dangerous. During a low blood sugar, you may shake, sweat, and feel disoriented. On the other hand, you may feel normal, although others around you may notice distinct changes in your personality and capabilities.

During a reaction, thinking becomes impaired due to lack of the glucose needed for the brain to function well. Although most organs can switch to fat or protein for fuel, glucose is the only fuel source for the brain. Loss of coordination, confusion, release of stress hormones, and irritability usually start when the blood sugar goes below 55 or 60 mg/dl (3.1 to 3.3 mmol), although these changes are not always recognized by the person having the reaction.

On an insulin pump, frequent readings below 50 mg/dl and nearly all readings below 40 mg/dl can be prevented. Regardless of how well you feel or think you feel, any blood sugar below 60 mg/dl (3.3 mmol) is an insulin reaction and can carry danger with it. A recent survey of over 2,000 pumpers in Germany showed that pumps can be very useful in avoiding reactions. Hospitalization for hypoglycemia among pumpers in this study occurred only once for every 16 years of use.

This chapter discusses the following aspects of insulin reactions:

- Causes
- Symptoms
- Treatment
- Prevention

137

Causes Of Insulin Reactions

Reactions are most likely to occur

1. When too much insulin is taken
2. When insulin is taken for a meal, but the meal is missed, delayed, or interrupted
3. When large or frequent boluses are used to bring down highs
4. After drinking alcohol
5. During and after exercise
6. On vacations, when stress is reduced and activity is often increased

Symptoms Of Insulin Reactions

Insulin reactions can occur with no symptoms, with only minor symptoms, or with full blown symptoms. Symptoms vary from person to person and also from one reaction to another. A reaction may be recognized first by the person having it or by others observing it.

Listed below are common symptoms of insulin reactions. Recognizing that an insulin reaction is underway allows early treatment. Be aware that symptoms may be harder to recognize when using an insulin pump. Due to precise insulin dosing with a pump, blood sugars often fall more gradually over time than with injections. Although this slower blood sugar drop provides more time to respond, it also can be associated with fewer symptoms. Learn to pay attention to and recognize these more subtle symptoms.

One or more of these symptoms can occur during any reaction. Some may never occur. Be sure to check your blood sugar at any time that you suspect a low blood sugar or anyone around you suspects one. If someone asks you to check your blood sugar, do so immediately and try to behave cooperatively.

> ## Symptoms For Insulin Reaction
> **You may experience any of these:**
> - sweating
> - shaking
> - irritability
> - blurred vision
> - fast heart rate
> - sudden tiredness
> - dizziness and confusion
> - numbness of the lips
> - nausea or vomiting
> - frequent sighing
> - headache
> - silliness
> - tingling

Blood sugar testing will alert you to insulin reactions you may be having with minimal symptoms or with minimal awareness of your symptoms. The faster you recognize a reaction, the faster you can respond and return to a normal blood sugar. A quick response also reduces stress hormone release and the chances of spiking afterward. When you see the results of a test, ask yourself if you have unused bolus insulin in your system. For instance, if your blood sugar is 120 mg/dl (6.7 mmol) two hours after a large bolus, you may want to eat at that time to avoid an approaching insulin reaction.

If it is available to you, continuous monitoring can alert you that a low blood sugar is approaching long before it occurs. Simply set the threshold of the monitor to give you a warning at an appropriate blood sugar reading and then act on the warning. Also pay attention to previous readings, or the trend in your blood sugar, to understand how fast your blood sugar is dropping, as well as what may have caused the high blood sugar in the first place, so you can avoid it the next time.

Nighttime Reactions

Night reactions are a special concern. More than 50% of severe insulin reactions occur at night. During sleep, early symptoms of low blood sugars go unrecognized, and even serious symptoms may not awaken you. If you wake up during the night with any of the symptoms below, check your blood sugar immediately. You may also eat quick-acting carbohydrate and then check.

Symptoms during the night may include

- Nightmares
- Waking up very alert or with a fast heart rate
- Damp night clothes, sheets, or pillow
- Restlessness and inability to go back to sleep
- Waking up with a feeling that something isn't right

Symptoms the next morning that may indicate a nighttime reaction include

- Waking up with a headache or "foggy-headed"
- Unusually high blood sugar after breakfast or before lunch
- A small amount of ketones but no glucose in the morning urine
- Loss of memory for words or names

If you have any of the nighttime symptoms, testing a 2 a.m. blood sugar for a few nights can do wonders in identifying and correcting this problem. Review possible causes and take action to avoid a reoccurrence.

> ### The First Rule of Good Control? Stop Your LOWS!
>
> When insulin reactions are frequent or severe, a major correction of basals and/or boluses is needed. After reducing your TDD, control should improve.
>
> A good place to begin is to reduce your TDD by 10 percent.

Daytime Lows

Because of Humalog's fast action, it is even more important to use fast carbs when treating lows. Fast carbs like glucose, jelly beans, or Gatorade work best to reverse the rapid drops that can be encountered with this insulin.

Those who use Regular insulin know they've really overdosed when a low blood sugar happens just two or three hours after a bolus. These lows require fast carbs followed by slow carbs, but lows that happen five or six hours after a bolus of Regular will not require as much carbohydrate to treat. Major lows with Humalog are most likely to happen within three hours of the bolus and need the treatment described in the previous paragraph. If the blood sugar goes low at three or more hours after a bolus, most of the last Humalog bolus is gone, and 10 to 15 grams of carbohydrate usually can remedy the problem.

Low blood sugars near bedtime also are easier to treat on Humalog. By bedtime, the action of the Humalog bolus taken for dinner is gone. Only a small amount of carbohydrate should be needed for a sound sleep if the night basal rate is correctly set. Under similar circumstances on Regular, both fast and slow carbohydrates would be needed to treat this low and prevent another one later during the night from that same dinner bolus of Regular.

How To Treat Your Insulin Reactions

Treat Quickly

Not even the most conscientious person can prevent every reaction, which means we all need to learn the best action for raising the blood sugar quickly to relieve symptoms and reduce aftereffects.

The best treatment for most lows, unless you will be having a meal right away, is a combination of simple and complex carbohydrates plus some protein. Ten to fifteen grams of quick carbohydrates, such as glucose, Sweet Tarts™ or honey will raise the blood sugar between 30 to 75 points (1.7 to 4.1 mmol) under most circumstances. Following this with a complex carb and protein can help keep the blood sugar from dropping too low again over the next several hours. As mentioned earlier, this second step may not be needed if the insulin you use is Humalog.

Treating insulin reactions with quick carbs returns your blood sugar to normal faster than eating or drinking anything else. Raising the low blood sugar quickly is important because fast action helps shut off the release of stress hormones. This will lower the chance of having a high blood sugar afterward, and it also improves your chances of recognizing the next reaction. You'll feel better if the body is quickly resupplied with the fuel it needs. Your brain, muscles and other cells will thank you. Remember that most cookies and candies do not act quickly enough.

Glucose, which is the sugar our blood sugar need; it may be referred to as dextrose on labels. It comes in tablets or candies like Sweet Tarts (see Table 15.1). These products quickly break down and reach the blood as 100 percent glucose; thus they are an excellent choice for raising blood sugars. Maltose, which is made of two glucose molecules, is also quite fast, but messy.

You need to know that table sugar is made from one glucose molecule plus one fructose molecule. When it breaks down in the stomach, only 50 percent is available immediately as glucose. Fruit juices, like orange juice, contain mostly fructose and are a poor choice for quick treatment of serious reactions because they take so long to raise the blood sugar. See the glycemic index on page 70 for more guidance as to the highest glycemic index foods, which most quickly raise the blood sugar.

How much glucose do you need? A good rule of thumb is that 1 gram of glucose raises the blood sugar 3, 4, or 5 points (for weights of 200 lb., 150 lb., and 100 lb. respectively). A 5 gram glucose tablet should raise your blood sugar between 15 and 25 points, depending on your weight and activity.

Table 15.1 Handy List Of Quick Carbs

Each has approx. 15 grams of carb:

- 1 tablespoon of molasses
- 3 BD or 4 generic glucose tablets
- 3 Smartie Rolls (3" cellophane rolls)
- 4 CanAm Dex4 glucose tablets
- 5 Dextrosols
- 6 SweetTart Packets (3 tabs/packet)
- 7 Pixy Stix
- 8 Sweet Tarts (3/4 in. - Lifesaver size)
- 14 Smarties (3/4 in. diameter roll)

Thanks to Laura Lyons, RN, CDE, for contributing this table.

Use 15 to 20 grams of quick carbohydrate for all low blood sugars. Check ahead of time to see how many grams of carbohydrate are in each glucose tablet you use to make sure you actually get 15 to 20 grams.

Table 15.1 lists a variety of quick carbohydrates. Each contains 15 grams of glucose or an equivalent sugar, and should raise the blood sugar rapidly between 45 and 75 points for people who weigh between 200 lb. and 100 lb., respectively. Test your blood sugar in 20 to 30 minutes after you treat the low to make sure that it has been corrected.

Remember that thinking and coordination remain abnormal for 30 minutes after the blood sugar has been brought back to normal. Wait 30 to 45 minutes after the blood sugar has returned to normal before driving a car or operating machinery.

Once you've eaten simple carbs that will raise the blood sugar quickly, consider your situation again. A recent bolus of insulin, extra exercise, or a missed meal all demand that more than 15 to 20 grams of carbs be taken. At bedtime, in particular, have an additional 10 grams or so of some carbohydrate lower on the glycemic index, such as a glass of milk or half an apple. Raw cornstarch, a complex carbohydrate that breaks down very slowly, is available in special bars to prevent overnight lows. An alternative to raw cornstarch is to have a high protein food, like cheese or peanut butter. If kidney disease is present, you need to subtract this protein from your allowed daily amount. Both proteins and complex carbohydrates help prevent the blood sugar from dropping for several hours.

Summary Of Treatment Plan For Typical Insulin Reactions

1. Eat 15 to 20 grams of quick-acting carbohydrates (Table 15.1).

2. Consider how long it is until your next meal and whether additional complex carbohydrates with protein are needed. If they are, add crackers and cheese or peanut butter, half an apple with cheese, or a cup of milk ten minutes after eating quick carbs.

3. Check to see whether any bolus insulin is still active, using the unused bolus rule in Chapter 13. Eat more carbs to compensate for any insulin still working.

4. Test the blood sugar again after 30 minutes to make sure it has risen. Repeat Step 1 if necessary.

5. Wait 30 to 45 minutes after the blood sugar has returned to normal before driving or operating machinery.

Don't Panic and Overeat

Panic attacks come from the release of stress hormones during lows. If you overdose on orange juice, chocolates, or the entire contents of your refrigerator, your goal of stable blood sugars becomes hard to achieve. If your blood sugars often go high after lows, you know you eat too much for your reactions. If you have frequent lows, your TDD is too high and this problem needs to be addressed as well.

Some people find themselves gaining weight from overtreating reactions, which is another reason to avoid panicking. Prepare for the panic by having a preset amount of quick carbohydrate handy at your bedside, in your pocket or purse, at your desk, in the glove compartment, and while exercising. Also memorize the fact that it takes only a little carb to counteract a low. A low doesn't mean unlimited treat time!

When treating an insulin reaction, it is important to look at how many hours have passed since the last bolus. If the last Humalog bolus was three or more hours ago, a small amount of carbohydrate should easily correct the low, assuming the basal rate is correctly set. If the insulin reaction occurs only an hour or two after the last bolus, much of that insulin has yet to act, and more carbohydrate than normal will be needed to treat this low. Of course, if you bolused 10 units of Humalog an hour ago in preparation for a meal and neglected eating the meal, a lot more than 15 or 20 grams of carbohydrate will be needed.

Prevent The Next Reaction

Keep in mind that one insulin reaction increases the risk of another. Researchers in Virginia found that the chance for having a second insulin reaction after an initial

> ### How To Prevent Lows
>
> - Test often.
>
> - Eat the meals and snacks that you've taken insulin for.
>
> - Count the carbohydrates in each meal and then match your carb bolus to them as well as to the current blood sugar.
>
> - Be careful drinking alcohol. Inebriation and hypoglycemia have a lot in common. Excess alcohol shuts off the glucose normally released from the liver and makes a low blood sugar likely.
>
> - Raise your premeal blood sugar target to 100 to 150 mg/dl (5.6 to 8.3 mmol) if you are having repeated lows.
>
> - Learn to use your test results to adjust your insulin doses and carbohydrates. For example, if low blood sugars occur in the afternoon, either an afternoon snack, a smaller bolus for lunch, or a lower basal rate in the afternoon can help avoid this problem.
>
> - Test often before, during, and after exercise. Exercise can lower the blood sugar for as long as 36 hours.
>
> - Always check blood sugars before driving and during long drives.

reaction increased to 46 percent in the next 24 hours, 24 percent on the second day, and 12 percent on the third day after the original reaction.[65] Some of this increased risk comes from an enhanced sensitivity to insulin that can occur following the first low blood sugar. A 10% lower temporary basal over the next 24 hours to avoid a second reaction may be wise. You might take other steps to keep your blood sugars higher for the next 24 hours, such as eating more carbs or lowering your carb boluses.

Not only is the risk of a second reaction higher, but symptoms during the second reaction become harder to recognize. When stress hormones are released during the first reaction, stores of these hormones, which create the warning signals, are reduced for the next two to three days.

How To Prevent Insulin Reactions

Recognize Trigger Situations

Be alert for changes in your daily routine (travel, vacation, weight loss, stress, etc.). These can all cause low blood sugars in some people.

Frequent or severe insulin reactions mean that too much insulin is being given. This is especially true if reactions occur within one to three hours after a bolus or if they require more than 15 grams of glucose to bring the blood sugar back to normal.

If either of these is happening to you, call your physician/health care team immediately to discuss lowering your basal rates and boluses.

Some people, particularly those who exercise strenuously or for prolonged periods, benefit from frequent basal and bolus adjustments to match changes in their activity level. More activity, less insulin. Less activity, more insulin. Almost everyone requires some periodic adjustments in their insulin doses, including the basal rate. Newer insulin pumps allow two or more different basal profiles that can be used on different days, as for exercise, weekends, or menses.

With experience, you will be making these changes as needed. Be sure to consult with your physician/health care team if you are uncertain what your own blood sugar results mean.

Insulin Reactions And Driving

Driving a car can be hypnotic or trancelike. With your attention on the road and other cars, you may not notice that your ability to think, to make decisions, and to interact with others has changed. If your blood sugar has been dropping slowly during a drive, a low blood sugar becomes especially hard to recognize. Don't drive if your blood sugar is below 80 mg/dl (5 mmol) before starting the car, or if it is likely to drop below 80 mg/dl (5 mmol) at any time during the drive.

The risk of injury or death to others and yourself is raised when you drive while low. If you are driving a car and become involved in an auto accident due to a low blood sugar, many states automatically suspend your license!

Always check your blood sugar before driving. Make sure you have glucose tablets or other quick carbohydrate easily accessible in your vehicle. Some people always eat some carbohydrate prior to driving, just to be safe. On the road, pull over and test your blood sugar if you have any doubts. On long drives, test every two hours. Don't be a statistic!

Severe Reactions

A severe reaction occurs whenever you are unable to handle the insulin reaction yourself. Situations in which a reaction become a concern involve being unable to react appropriately while driving, or losing consciousness completely, or suffering convulsions. For severe situations like these, glucagon is always the best treatment. Glucagon is another hormone made by the pancreas, which rapidly raises the blood sugar by triggering a release of glucose stored within the liver. An injection of glucagon is a sure way to raise very low blood sugars quickly.

Glucagon can be used when someone is unconscious or having seizures due to hypoglycemia, when a person is resisting treatment due to hypoglycemia unawareness, when an illness keeps someone from eating to correct a low blood sugar, or when nausea prevents eating to correct a low.

Glucagon kits are available by prescription and should be kept at home by everyone on insulin. They can be stored at room temperature or in the refrigerator and are stable for several years after purchase, but dating should be checked periodically to ensure potency.

Someone who is likely to be available during an insulin reaction should be instructed by a Certified Diabetes Educator, a trained nurse, or a pharmacist on how to inject glucagon. The person with diabetes may need to give herself/himself a glucagon injection at times, such as when a carb bolus has been taken but nausea prevents eating. They typical dose within the glucagon syringe is 1 mg. of glucagon and this is often more than is needed to correct a low. One half a dose is usually all that's required for an adult or child. If needed, the other half dose can be given ten minutes later.

What The Person With Diabetes Can Do

Avoiding low blood sugars through careful management of insulin doses and carbohydrate intake is always the best strategy. Even with the best of efforts, hypoglycemia can happen occasionally. When a low blood sugar does occur, the following tips can help in treating it quickly and effectively:

- Always carry with you quick carbs like glucose tablets or simple sugar candies to eat when you suspect a low or a low occurs.

- Assume the primary responsibility for handling your own low blood sugars.

- Be willing to accept help from others. Let family and friends know about your diabetes and what they can do to help.

- Be more careful of lows when changing your insulin doses, food choices, and activity. Test more often during these times.

- Let family and friends know when you have become more vulnerable to lows because you are varying your regimen or life style. Share what is happening with your blood sugar control so that others can help you.

- Keep glucagon available at home for severe lows. Be sure that a family member or a friend has been well-trained in how and when to inject it.

- Be especially careful if lows are happening frequently since this is a major cause of hypoglycemia unawareness.

How Others Can Help

By recognizing what is happening and taking appropriate action, other people can help someone suffering from hypoglycemia unawareness avoid a severe reaction. If the actions of someone who takes insulin become unusual over a short period of time (usually 10 to 30 minutes), an insulin reaction is the likely cause.

Irrational thought, anger, irritability, running away, or insistence that "I feel fine" may occur. Thinking is impaired, fight-or-flight hormone levels are high, and an emotional response is likely. Hypoglycemia unawareness may be occurring if the person refuses to acknowledge a problem. Gentle coaxing and encouragement often can help convince the person with hypoglycemia unawareness to eat or drink fast-acting carbohydrate. Remember that confronting someone who is not thinking clearly and has a high level of stress hormones is not wise.

One way to deal with future episodes of hypoglycemia unawareness is to agree on a plan of action ahead of time. The person with diabetes can agree to test the blood sugar or eat if a supportive coworker or family member request this, perhaps with a discreet signal. If needed, glucagon can be given by injection by a trained family member, a friend, or even by the affected person to raise the blood sugar rapidly.

If you have ever become unconscious or incoherent due to a low blood sugar and required assistance to treat it, discuss this thoroughly with your physician as soon as possible. You are likely to benefit from working with a physician who understands and specializes in insulin delivery to avoid repeating this dangerous situation.

Many problems associated with hypoglycemia are caused when the person experiencing it cannot think clearly. The brain works only on glucose as fuel. The ability to think, reason, and solve problems becomes more and more impaired as the blood sugar drops to lower and lower levels. People vary in how they experience a low blood sugar, and how they may act during any particular low blood sugar also varies tremendously.

Anger during a low blood sugar usually is triggered by the release of stress hormones. Normally, the release of these hormones will help return the blood sugar levels to normal, but these "fight or flight" hormones and the associated hypoglycemia also have a darker side that makes it harder for a person to react in a normal way. It helps for others to recognize as early as possible that a low blood sugar is taking place so that it may be treated quickly.

Tips For Helpers

At times it may be difficult to assist someone who is having a low blood sugar because the low causes irrational, confused, or angry behavior. These tips may help under those circumstances.

- Control your own emotions first. If the person you are attempting to help is stubborn, acts silly or becomes angry, don't take this personally. Prepare your own mind to deal with the variety of hypoglycemia attitudes you may encounter.

- Take charge of the situation. Use a gentle but firm tone. A nonconfrontational stance, such as sitting or standing beside the person, helps.

- Say, "Here, have this piece of candy." or "I'm going to drink a coke (take a drink yourself), here, have a sip." or "I think you need to eat (drink) this."

- Avoid direct questions like "Are you low?", "Do you need to test?", or "Do you need to eat?" The person who is unable to think clearly may find "NO" the most convenient answer.

- Don't let the person drive a car, run machinery, or become involved in other dangerous activities that require coordination.

- Ask for help from others whenever needed. Keep embarrassment to a minimum and the person's cooperation to a maximum.

Opportunity is missed by most people because it is dressed in overalls and looks like work.

Thomas Edison

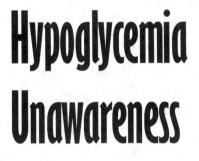

CHAPTER 16

Hypoglycemia Unawareness

Research is bringing relief for people who have one of the most distressing problems of diabetes. The problem, called hypoglycemia unawareness, occurs when a person has problems treating his own low blood sugar because he is unaware he is having a severe low. A person with hypoglycemia unawareness has lost some or all of the warning symptoms of lows and cannot recognize a low blood sugar without testing.

A person with normal responses usually feels and can act on the basis of warning symptoms of lows, like the shaking and sweating caused by the release of counter-regulatory stress hormones. The person with hypoglycemia unawareness has lost rational thought processes before any hypoglycemia symptoms are recognized. Having diabetes with frequent lows for many years often causes reduced stress hormone release, and this results in symptoms that are mild and hard to recognize. That hypoglycemia unawareness could occur during sleep is not surprising, but it also occurs in some people while they are awake.

Luckily, even though a person may not recognize a low, automatic responses usually cause enough counter-regulatory hormones to be released so that the liver eventually raises the glucose levels. If these hormones are depleted, however, the automatic responses may not work. Women may be more prone to this problem than men because of reduced counter-regulatory responses and reduced symptoms.[68] Unless recognized and treated by someone else, the low may create serious problems, including grand mal seizures. If you've ever witnessed seizure activity or bizarre behavior in someone else, you have some idea of the seriousness of this problem and its danger.

Hypoglycemia unawareness is not rare. The major counter-regulatory hormone that causes glucose release by the liver to raise the blood sugar is glucagon. Glucagon secretion usually is reduced in most people who have Type 1 diabetes within the first two to ten years after onset. Hypoglycemia unawareness occurs in 17 percent of those with Type 1 diabetes. The risk is far lower in people with Type 2 diabetes because their low blood sugars are infrequent. A study of tight control in Type 2 diabetes done by the Veterans Administration showed that severe reactions occurred only four percent as often in Type 2 as compared to Type 1.[69] An insulin reaction can occur in Type 2 only if the person uses insulin, a sulfonylurea, or Prandin™.

The lower a person's average blood sugar, the higher their risk for hypoglycemia unawareness. Hypoglycemia unawareness was three times as common in the intensively controlled group compared to the conventionally controlled group in the Diabetes Control and Complications Trial, with 55 percent of these episodes occurring during sleep. On the other hand, in a study of adolescents by Yale University researchers, a group of 25 teens on pumps was able to obtain lower HbA1c values after 12 months, 7.5% versus 8.3%, and also reduce their risk of severe hypoglycemia by 50% compared to another 50 teens using multiple daily injections.[70]

What Causes Hypoglycemia Unawareness?

Situations that can trigger hypoglycemia unawareness include:

- Frequent low blood sugars
- A rapid drop in the blood sugar
- Having diabetes for many years
- Stress or depression
- Situations where self-care is a low priority
- Alcohol consumption in the last 12 hours
- An insulin reaction in the last 24 to 48 hours
- Certain medications like beta blockers

Reaction symptoms may become less obvious after having diabetes for several years because the body begins to release less of the hormones like epinephrine and glucagon that typically cause sweating and shaking. Drinking alcohol can contribute to hypoglycemia unawareness because the mind becomes less capable of recognizing what's happening, the liver is blocked from creating glucose needed to raise the blood sugar, and the release of free fatty acids (the backup to glucose for fuel) is also blocked.[71]

Frequent low blood sugars appear to be the major culprit in hypoglycemia unawareness. The way a person loses warning signals after a low blood sugar was demonstrated in research by Dr. Thiemo Veneman and other researchers.[72] Dr. Veneman and his group had 10 people who did not have diabetes spend a day at the hospital on two occasions. While they slept, the researchers used insulin to lower their blood sugars to between 40 and 45 mg/dl (2.2 to 2.5 mmol) for two hours in the middle of the night. (No, they didn't wake up! People don't wake up during most nighttime reactions. They actually remember only the reactions during which they wake up.) Five people went through a nighttime low on the first visit and the other five on the second visit. On waking in the morning, all were given insulin to lower their blood sugars to see at what point they would recognize symptoms of low blood sugars.

Dr. Veneman found that after sleeping through a reaction at night, people had far more trouble recognizing a low blood sugar the following day. The warning symptoms are vague because counter-regulatory hormones, like epinephrine, norepinephrine, and glucagon are released more slowly and in smaller concentrations following a reaction that occurred during the previous 24 hours. In other words, a recent low blood sugar depletes a person without diabetes of the hormones that provide an alert for the reaction and makes it more likely the person will fail to recognize a second low. It's even more likely that this sequence of events would cause hypoglycemia unawareness in a person with diabetes.

How To Stop Hypoglycemia Unawareness

The major cause of hypoglycemia unawareness is frequent low blood sugars. Research has shown that some people who have hypoglycemia unawareness can regain the symptoms of reactions by avoiding frequent lows.[73] Preventing all lows resulted in increased symptoms of low blood sugars after only 2 weeks and a return to nearly normal symptoms after 3 months. In this study, Dr. Carmine Fanelli and other researchers in Rome reduced the frequency of insulin reactions in people who had diabetes for seven years or less and who suffered from hypoglycemia unawareness. The subjects raised the target for their premeal blood sugars to 140 mg/dl (7.8 mmol) and the frequency of hypoglycemia dropped from once every other day to once every 22

days. Because the higher premeal blood sugars led to fewer insulin reactions, people regained the ability to recognize low blood sugar symptoms.

The counter-regulatory hormone response in these subjects, which alerts them to the presence of a low blood sugar, returned to values that were nearly

> ### How To Stop Hypoglycemia Unawareness
>
> If you suffer from hypoglycemia unawareness, aim for higher blood sugars, so that you prevent all lows. Stay above 60 mg/dl or 70 mg/dl (3.3 to 3.9 mmol) **at all times**. Set your premeal targets at 100 mg/dl to 180 mg/dl (5.6 to 10 mmol), and carefully discuss how to achieve this range with your physician. Lower your TDD, give smaller carb and high blood sugar boluses, and use at least 50% of your TDD as basal.

normal. These researchers demonstrated that hypoglycemia unawareness is reversible.

What are the best ways to avoid lows in order to reverse hypoglycemia unawareness? You can start by keeping your blood sugar target slightly higher, matching insulin doses closely to your diet and exercise, and using special care following a first reaction. Consider a blood sugar below 60 mg/dl (3.3 mmol) a serious reaction and practice avoiding it.

You can also consider using the medication Precose (acarbose), which delays the absorption of carbohydrates. This has been shown to decrease the risk of insulin reactions. Precose can be combined with a modest lowering of carbohydrate boluses. Also be quick to correct problems that arise from stress, depression, or other self-care causes. Be especially careful when drinking alcohol. Limit consumption to one or two drinks per day to avoid shutting off the liver's response. For people with a physically active lifestyle, insulin adjustments may be needed every day to match variability.

If insulin reactions occur frequently or if an episode of hypoglycemia unawareness occurs, insulin doses must be lowered immediately. An occasional 2 a.m. blood test can do wonders in preventing hypoglycemia unawareness due to unrecognized nighttime reactions. Using current or soon to be available continuous interstitial glucose measuring devices can alert you and your health care team to occurrences of unrecognized hypoglycemia. These devices allow rapid basal and bolus changes to prevent reoccurrence. With an appropriate lower threshold alarm, you can be warned of any blood sugar that drops to this threshold level.

Can a person who has had diabetes for many years reverse hypoglycemia unawareness? Although research provides conflicting results, anecdotal information suggests that improved control enables even people with long-term diabetes to regain more symptoms of their insulin reactions. Avoiding lows always seems to reduce the risk of hypoglycemia unawareness.

As devices that allow continuous monitoring become available, wearing a monitor at all times will eliminate hypoglycemia unawareness and most episodes of hypoglycemia entirely. Another alternative would be the short-term use of one of these devices to break the cycle of lows, allow better basal and bolus adjustments, and allow recovery of hypoglycemia symptoms.

Call your doctor immediately if you need assistance for any low blood sugar. If it happens once, it's likely to happen again. Discuss how to make immediate bolus and basal adjustments to avoid a reoccurrence.

People tell me one thing and out the other.
I feel as much like I did yesterday as I did today.
I never liked room temperature.
My throat is closer than it seems....
I don't like any of my loved ones.

Daniel M. Wegner's reading test for brain damage

CHAPTER 17

Severe Highs and Ketoacidosis

Severe high blood sugars and ketoacidosis (DKA) are serious medical problems that sometimes occur in diabetes. These life-threatening conditions are most often seen in Type 1 or insulin-dependent diabetes because little to no insulin is produced. Severe high blood sugars, usually accompanied by ketoacidosis, are often present when a person is first diagnosed with Type 1 diabetes.

High blood sugars and ketoacidosis can be triggered in people with Type 1 diabetes by bad insulin, a severe infection, a severe illness, a pump problem, or simply forgetting to take insulin. They can also occur in people with Type 2 diabetes under the stress of a severe illness like pneumonia or a heart attack. In children and adolescents with Type 1 diabetes, ketoacidosis can be triggered by normal growth spurts that increase the body's need for more insulin. When an infection or illness is causing the problem, high blood sugars will be difficult to bring down until the underlying problem is dealt with.

High blood sugars can exist for some time without triggering ketoacidosis. Ketoacidosis begins only after insulin levels in the body go very low. When insulin is low, glucose cannot be used as fuel. Glucose is the body's first choice for energy, but if the glucose in the blood can't enter the cells due to lack of insulin, the body must start burning fat even though glucose is quite high in the blood.

Burning fat might at first sound like a good thing, especially if you are trying to lose weight, but burning excessive fat turns out to be quite unhealthy. When ketones, a normal by-product of fat metabolism, are produced at high levels, the blood becomes highly acidic causing nausea and vomiting. The vomiting, combined with high blood sugars, leads to rapid dehydration. An acidic blood condition complicated by severe dehydration is quite serious and frequently leads to death.

Any time that insulin delivery is interrupted on a pump, the risk for ketoacidosis is present. The small reservoir of active insulin in the body disappears over three to five hours. Blood sugars start to rise within 90 minutes after insulin delivery is disrupted. In seven research studies done since 1985 on DKA in pumpers, ketoacidosis occurred on average once for every 16 years of use. Of course, the risk of ketoacidosis can be reduced greatly by using proper pump techniques. Check your blood sugar often once you realize that it is climbing, and start treating immediately. This includes giving insulin by syringe until the cause for poor control is identified and corrected.

When continuous monitoring is used, and a threshold set for a warning alarm at an appropriate high reading, high blood sugars will not exist for hours without detection. Ketoacidosis, which requires high blood sugars for several hours, becomes unlikely, unless the cause is a severe illness, or insulin delivery from the pump is interrupted and the user continues trying to give boluses, not recognizing that insulin is no longer being given.

Symptoms And Testing

Early symptoms of ketoacidosis include tiredness, great thirst, frequent urination, dry skin, a fruity odor to the breath, abdominal pain, and nausea. Advanced symptoms include vomiting, shortness of breath, and rapid breathing

Check For Ketones:

- for any unexplained high blood sugar
- whenever a blood sugar is above 300 mg/dl (16.7 mmol)
- if a fruity odor is detected on the breath
- if abdominal pain is present
- if nausea or vomiting occurs
- if you are breathing rapidly and short of breath.

If a moderate or large amount of ketones register on the test strip, ketoacidosis is present and treatment is required immediately.

as the body tries to clear the bloodstream of ketones and high blood sugars. These symptoms are due to ketone poisoning and should never be ignored. As soon as a person begins to vomit or has difficulty breathing, immediate treatment in an emergency room is required to prevent coma and possible death.

Everyone with diabetes needs to know how to recognize and treat ketoacidosis. Ketones travel from the blood into the urine and can be detected in the urine with ketone test strips available at any pharmacy. Always keep ketone strips on hand but store them in a dry area and replace them as soon as they are outdated.

New meters like the Precision Xtra™, can measure blood sugar but also have the ability to measure blood ketone levels. This ability to measure blood ketones offers a tremendous advantage for pump users. A pumper who finds his blood sugar is unexpectedly 300 mg/dl (16.7 mmol) would want to measure his blood ketone level. If ketones are normal, a simple bolus should correct the problem. However, if ketone levels are high in this situation, the pumper would take Humalog by injection and change out their entire infusion set because insulin delivery appears to have failed.

Measuring ketones in the blood allows ketoacidosis to be detected at least two to four hours earlier than waiting for ketones to show up in the urine. It also allows home treatment with insulin and hydration to be evaluated for effectiveness much faster than waiting for ketone levels to drop slowly in the urine.

Treatment

Drink lots of fluid to correct dehydration. Dehydration is caused by excess urination from the high blood sugars and can worsen quickly if vomiting begins.

During ketoacidosis, staying hydrated is IMPORTANT. Drink lots of fluids.

What To Do If You Have Ketoacidosis

- Check your blood sugar hourly until control has been regained.

- Drink a large amount of water, noncaloric or low caloric fluids immediately, and continue with 8 to 12 oz. every 30 minutes. Water with Nu-Salt™, Gatorade, and similar fluids are good because they help restore potassium levels.

- Take Humalog by injection at least every 3 hours, using a new bottle of insulin, until blood sugars are below 200 mg/dl (11 mmol). Your normal doses for high blood sugars may need to be increased by 50 to 200 percent, and if an infection or other major illness is causing your highs, more insulin than this will be needed.

- If nausea starts, call your physician.

- If vomiting starts or you are unable to drink fluids, call your physician and go to an emergency room immediately.

When an infection or illness is causing the problem, high blood sugars will be difficult to bring down until the underlying problem is dealt with. If nausea or vomiting keep you from drinking fluids, call your physician and immediately go to an emergency room for treatment.

Any occurrence of a severe high or ketoacidosis should raise a red flag. The absence of a clear reason, such as illness or infection, may indicate that the pump has run dry, is leaking, or has clogged. It may also indicate that the insulin is bad, the basal rates or boluses are incorrect, or the basic principles of blood sugar control are not understood. Be sure to discuss any problems you have regarding high blood sugars or ketoacidosis with your physician so that problems can be resolved quickly and prevented from happening again.

Table 17.1 Steps To Prevent And Treat Ketoacidosis On A Pump

Anytime you have an unexplained high blood sugar, or with any reading over 300 mg/dl (16.7 mmol) on an insulin pump, suspect an insulin delivery problem. If there is a clear reason for the high reading, take a bolus and recheck your sugar in one hour to ensure it is being corrected.

If there is no clear reason for the high, or the second blood sugar remains high:
1. Check for pump or site-related problems (Chapters 22 and 23).
2, Check your blood or urine for ketones.

If ketones are OK*:	If ketones are HIGH**:
1. Give a normal bolus with the pump 2. Test your blood sugar again in one hour. If your sugar is not lower in one hour, follow the procedure to the right. 3. If lower at one hour, recheck in another one to two hours and use the unused bolus rule (Chapter 13) at that time to determine if an additional high blood sugar bolus is needed. 4. If your blood sugar remains high or ketones appear, call your physician and follow the procedure to the right.	1. Ketones suggest you have a problem with insulin delivery from your pump or a serious illness. If you have any reason to suspect an illness, **call your physician**. 2. Correct the high sugar with **injected insulin** from a syringe or pen. More insulin than normal may be required, especially if ketones have been present for several hours, or if an illness is causing the problem. 3. Start by drinking water or water with a pinch of Nu-Salt™ until **well-hydrated**. Then drink 8 to 12 ounces of fluid every hour until control is regained. 4. Replace the insulin cartridge and entire infusion set, using a new site. 5. Test your blood sugar in two hours. If it is not lower, call your physician immediately. 6. If your sugar is lower at two hours, use the unused bolus rule (Chapter 13) to determine if an additional high blood sugar bolus is needed. 7. If your blood sugar remains high, or nausea worsens, call your physician. 8. If vomiting begins at any time, **go immediately to the nearest ER** for IV hydration and further testing.

* OK = urine ketones are negative or small, or blood ketones are less than 0.6 mmol/L
** HIGH = urine ketones are moderate or high, or blood ketones are above 0.6 mmol/L

Thanks to Geri Wood, RN, BSN, CDE and John Stanchfield, MD, of Salt Lake City for their suggestions.

If at first you don't succeed, find out if the loser gets anything.

Bill Lyon

Exercise

"The only reason I would take up jogging is so I could hear heavy breathing again," said the late columnist Erma Bombeck. People with diabetes will be happy to know there are even better reasons to exercise.

This chapter explains exercise's

- Benefits
- Risks
- Effect on blood sugar and insulin
- Propensity to cause insulin reactions and how to avoid them

Benefits

Exercise sharpens the mind and tones the body. It makes the heart stronger and the lungs more efficient. It increases endurance and resistance to stress and fatigue. It combats depression and creates a sense of well-being. Exercise helps lower body fat and cholesterol readings. In fact, not exercising is as much a risk factor for heart disease as smoking a pack of cigarettes a day!

In a study of Harvard alumni, researchers found that the human lifespan increases steadily as exercise levels rise from burning 500 calories a week (couch potato) to 3,500 calories per week (physically fit).[74] The exercise needed to burn 3,500 calories is equivalent to walking three miles an hour for seven hours a week, bicycling 10 miles an hour for five hours a week, or running nine miles an hour for 2.7 hours a week. As you can see, the more intense the exercise, the less time you need to spend doing it. All of these forms of exercise provide benefit, with aerobic exercise providing the greatest amount of all. See Table 18.1 for more guidance.

It appears that even moderate levels of exercise done regularly will protect the heart. If you think burning 3,500 calories each week is too much, try doing moderate exercise regularly. Brisk walking or bicycling for 30 minutes five days a week has been shown to help prevent heart disease and increase lifespan.[74] This level of exercise uses 1,000 calories a week and appears to have major benefits for the heart. That is helpful news if you find brisk walking more appealing and safer than running marathons.

Risks

Along with numerous benefits, exercise also creates some risks. Always discuss exercise plans with your physician/health care team before starting. This is especially true if you've had diabetes a long time or have any diabetes-related problems, like nerve damage, eye changes, kidney disease, or a history of heart or blood vessel problems.

Blood flow and blood pressure both increase during exercise, which allow increased amounts of oxygen and fuel to reach the muscles. Blood flow may increase by as much as 15 or 20 times above normal resting levels during strenuous exercise. This possibly increased blood flow and pressure could harm organs and blood vessels weakened by past high blood sugars or could place extra strain on the heart. Such risks have to be considered before beginning an exercise program, especially ones like weight lifting or scuba diving, which can raise the blood pressure significantly. A more gradual increase in training level may be required if blood vessel damage is a concern.

If you have any nerve damage, you face some special challenges. Nerve damage can reduce your ability to sense pain and increase risk of injury to insensitive feet. Don't avoid exercise. Rather, choose the type and level of exercise you do carefully in order to protect your feet. For instance, swimming or biking may be a better choice than jogging.

Autonomic neuropathy, which is damage to nerves that control processes like digestion, heart rate, and blood vessel tone, can create an artificially low heart rate and

Table 18.1 Let Your Goal Determine How You Exercise			
Your Goal	**Frequency**	**Intensity**	**Duration**
Reduce Risk of Heart Disease and Illness	2-3 X a week	40% max. heart rate	15-30 min.
Get Physically Fit	4 X a week	70-90% max. heart rate	15-30 min.
Lose Weight	5 X a week	45-60% max. heart rate	45-60 min.
Use this formula to determine your maximum heart rate: 220 - your age = your maximum heart rate			

interfere with blood flow to exercising muscles. Autonomic neuropathy also carries with it a higher risk for heart disease. A heart rate monitor may not be an accurate way to measure exercise intensity in those with this condition. A more gradual training program under supervision is strongly advised when autonomic neuropathy is present. This type of neuropathy can be detected with an EKG or by measuring the change in blood pressure as you go from a reclining to a standing position.

Dehydration is a major concern for any athlete. Staying hydrated is essential for turning glucose and fat into energy. Dehydration can create confusion and impair thinking, which makes distinguishing between it and a low blood sugar difficult. Dehydration becomes more likely as blood sugars rise, especially if they are combined with hot weather. Frequent intake of fluid before, during, and after exercise is essential to preventing dehydration and loss of energy.

How Your Blood Sugar Affects Your Exercise

As shown in Table 18.3, normal blood sugars during exercise allow the muscles and heart to receive glucose and fat as fuel in amounts that allow maximum performance. For the athlete with diabetes, performance suffers when the blood sugar goes high or low. For optimum performance, an athlete must judge accurately how to replace the carbs burned and how to adjust insulin doses to ensure an ideal flow of fuels. Insulin controls the availability of glucose and fat as fuels. This is critical for maximum performance.

Even the amount of oxygen we breath depends on blood sugar control. Research from Austria shows that air flow to the lungs is reduced as much as 15 percent when blood sugars run high.[75] This oxygen deficit caused by high blood sugars can also impair athletic performance.

Table 18.2 Easy Way To Determine Heart Rate

Feel your pulse at the wrist, and count your pulse for 10 seconds, then use this table to find beats per minute.

10 Second Pulse Count	Beats Per Minute
10	60
11	66
12	72
13	78
14	84
15	90
16	96
17	102
18	108
19	114
20	120
21	126
22	132
23	138
24	144
25	150
26	156
27	162
28	168
29	174
30	180

How You Get Fuel For Exercise

When travelling by car, you can easily determine how much gasoline is needed for a trip. Once you decide how long a trip will take (duration), the car's speed (effort or intensity), and the miles per gallon the car gets at that speed, you can calculate the number of gallons of gasoline (energy) needed. If you put this amount of fuel in the gas tank before the trip, you won't run out of gas.

Estimating fuel needed for exercise, with diabetes, is similar. If someone weighs 150 pounds and runs 30 minutes (duration) at seven miles per hour (effort or intensity), he or she can determine the amount of energy, about 320 calories in this case, that will be used in the run.

The human body is different from a car engine, however, in that it can use various fuels. Internal stores of both glucose and fat, as well as carbs recently eaten, can be used as fuel. Insulin orchestrates the availability of glucose and fat stores to match the intensity and duration of various activities. For that reason, both the insulin level in the blood and the intake of carbohydrate must be controlled. This will keep the blood sugar normal throughout the workout.

A simple way to keep blood sugars normal when exercising with diabetes is to eat extra carbohydrate. This method helps maintain body weight and works very well for exercise that lasts less than 45 minutes.

Table 18.3 How Your Blood Sugar Affects Performance

Blood Sugar	How Sugar And Insulin Affect Metabolism	Impact On Performance
< 65 mg/dl	Too much insulin and not enough glucose available to cells	Tiredness, poor performance
65 to 180	Efficient fuel flow	Maximum performance
> 180 mg/dl	Glucose less able to enter muscle cells if insulin level is low, but will come down if insulin OK	Performance may be reduced
> 250 mg/dl	If insulin level is OK, blood sugars come down	Performance lower, exercise OK to do
> 250 mg/dl	If insulin level is TOO LOW, blood sugars will rise higher	Tiredness and poor performance. Check for ketones, take insulin before exercise

Since carbohydrate is the nutrient most important to performance, some intake of carbohydrate during longer exercise also is required. If you know how many carbohydrates are consumed in a particular exercise, you can eat foods containing that same number of carbs to maintain control. If an activity is longlasting, a reduction in insulin doses will likely be needed.

The first fuel source tapped when you start moderate or strenuous exercise is the glucose already present in the blood. This limited supply is rapidly followed by the release of glycogen stores from larger stores in muscle and liver. Although glucose and glycogen are easily accessible and rapidly released, the body's total supply is limited. For instance during strenuous exercise, glucose in the bloodstream can be depleted in only four minutes, compared to 30 minutes at rest.[76] The liver plays the most critical role in supplying glucose for exercise through its conversion of stored glycogen for release as glucose into the bloodstream. These stores, too, can be quickly depleted within the first 20 to 30 minutes of very strenuous exercise. It is also important to note that insulin levels must be low to access these internal glycogen stores.

Body fat acts as your largest source of fuel during exercise. Fat stores are about 2,000 times as large as the glucose supply in the blood and provide our greatest quick source of energy. These stores are nearly impossible to deplete, but again a reduced insulin level is needed for full access to them.

ExCarbs, or Exercise Carbs, is a system that measures the impact exercise will have on the blood sugar and provides options to use for maintaining control. It can help you increase carb intake precisely or reduce insulin doses to balance various types of exercise. ExCarbs can be eaten to replace the carbohydrate consumed during physical activity.; no carb boluses are taken to compensate for these carbs because they are used to replace some of the carbs consumed during exercise. ExCarbs also can be used to guide insulin dose reductions. How to use ExCarbs is covered in the next chapter.

Carb Loading

To improve performance, many athletes "fuel up" the glycogen stores in muscle cells by eating diets high in carbohydrate. Called "carb loading", this is often done just prior to major exercise events. Diets low in carbohydrate rob muscles of the glycogen stores they need for maximum endurance and performance.

For example, a trained marathon runner on a high carb diet can run for about four hours before exhaustion sets in, but when eating food that is high in fat or protein, and low in carbohydrate, the same athlete will become exhausted in less than an hour and a half, long before a marathon could be completed. Although fat and protein can act as fuels during exercise, endurance suffers if these nutrients replace the carbohydrate required to build muscle glycogen.

What Effect Does Your Insulin Level Have On Your Performance?

The amount of insulin in your blood determines how much carbohydrate and fat you are able to use as fuel, as well as where the fuel has to come from. It is important to remember that both too much or too little insulin in the blood can cause severe fuel delivery problems.

For the nondiabetic, these problems never occur because the body automatically makes rapid changes in the blood insulin level. At the start of a strenuous exercise like running a marathon, the blood insulin level will drop to half of its pre-exercise level in the first 15 minutes.[77] With moderate exercise, about an hour passes before the same drop in the blood insulin level is seen.

This drop in the insulin level as exercise begins allows

- glucose to be released from glycogen stores in the muscle and liver
- fat to be released and used as fuel, and
- new glucose to be created by the liver (a minor contribution).

A drop in the insulin level allows cells to switch gradually from glucose to fat as their primary fuel as an activity continues, instead of depending on much smaller supplies of glucose. The blood sugar remains steadier when muscles can access internal glycogen and fat stores.

Accessing stored fat as fuel becomes more important as the length of exercise extends to 40 or 60 minutes and longer. When insulin levels are lowered, the risk of a low blood sugar is reduced because fat stores can be tapped more easily for energy. When your insulin level is lower, you can exercise longer with less danger of a low

Table 18.4 How Your Insulin Level Affects Performance			
Insulin Level	Effect on Stress Hormones	Effect on Glucose and Fat	Effect on Performance
Low	Increased	Less glucose enters muscles, more glucose and fat are released into blood	Blood sugar usually high, poor performance, possible ketosis
Ideal	Normal	Glucose enters muscles, glucose and fat are released as fuel normally	Normal blood sugar and optimal performance
High	Decreased, until hypoglycemia begins	Increased glucose entry into muscles, reduced release of glucose and fat from internal stores	Blood sugar usually low, poor performance

blood sugar. Although insulin levels in diabetes do not adjust automatically for exercise, you can set your own insulin level with a pump to match the intensity and duration of any type of exercise.

What happens, though, if your basals and boluses are not adjusted appropriately? If insulin levels are too high, more sugar enters exercising muscles from the blood, while less sugar is released from glycogen stores and less fat is available to replace glucose. The blood sugar drops rapidly into an insulin reaction unless the blood sugar was high at the start of exercise or carbs are eaten during the exercise.

On the other hand, if blood insulin levels drop too low, more glucose and free fatty acids are released into the blood, and the glucose in the blood is less able to enter exercising muscles. Blood sugars then rise. Table 18.4 shows some of the effects the insulin level has on blood sugar levels, stress hormone levels, and fuel metabolism.

If your blood sugar is 250 mg/dl (13.9 mmol) or above, exercise often is not recommended because the insulin level may be dangerously low. Although your insulin level cannot be tested directly, in certain situations you can accurately guess that it's low. For instance, if your blood sugar was good at bedtime and you ate no bedtime snack but

High Blood Sugar Versus Dehydration

A high blood sugar during or after exercise can be caused by too little insulin, but it can also be triggered by dehydration. If you think your insulin is adequate and your pump is working but you're thirsty and your blood sugar is unusually high, try drinking three to six 8 oz. glasses of water or other noncaloric liquid.

Test again in 30 minutes to see if your blood sugar has come down. If it hasn't returned to a normal range, take an injection of insulin to bring it down if you have any doubt about your pump's operation. Otherwise, bolus.

If you are only dehydrated, drinking liquids will bring the blood sugar down some or all the way. Of course, the best way to avoid dehydration is to drink extra water whenever you exercise and to drink long before you get thirsty.

your reading the next morning when you awaken is 200 mg/dl (11.1 mmol) or higher, you know your insulin level is low. Exercising under these circumstances can cause a further rise in your blood sugar level, unless you bolus before starting.

Contrast this to a situation in which an athlete intentionally raises her blood sugar above 250 as she prepares for a long athletic event. By lowering her carb bolus and eating extra carbs before the event starts, she can start the event confidently because a quick drop in blood sugar will be seen shortly after she starts exercising. Even though her blood sugar is high, she has enough insulin in her system to lower it as the glucose moves from the blood into exercising muscles. Of course, no test can tell you your insulin level so you must test your blood sugar at hourly intervals for a couple of times of trying this and any time you are in doubt.

An alternative to raising the blood sugar so high intentionally is to reduce both bolus and basal insulin sufficiently so that less carbohydrate has to be eaten before the event in order to exercise safely. With a lower insulin level, less carbohydrate is needed at the start of the event. Therefore, the blood sugar does not rise so high. In addition, less carbohydrate is needed during the event to prevent an insulin reaction because insulin levels have been lowered and internal glycogen stores are more accessible.

Stress Hormones And Exercise

Another example demonstrates the importance of the insulin level. During very strenuous, anaerobic exercise, like running the 100-yard dash or power weight-lifting, glucose provides almost all of the fuel required in the event. A very rapid release of glucose into the blood occurs from glycogen stores, driven by rising stress hormone levels. A similar rise occurs at the start of competitive aerobic events where rising stress hormone levels cause a large glucose release from glycogen stores.

> **Remember: Your blood sugar control during exercise depends on**
>
> - Your current insulin level
> - Your current blood sugar
> - Your training level
> - The length and intensity of the activity
> - Your stress hormone levels
> - Any recent low blood sugars

This stress-released glucose must be moved rapidly into exercising muscle to keep the blood sugar from rising. To enable a fast transfer of large amounts of glucose, the body of a person without diabetes quickly increases their blood insulin level rather than lowering it. Someone with diabetes is less able to do this because external insulin delivery, even from a pump, cannot respond this quickly to raise the insulin level.

Therefore, a sizable rise in the blood sugar is seen following very strenuous events, even though the person starts with a normal blood sugar. To prevent this from happening, a small bolus may be given prior to very strenuous exercise so that the blood sugar won't rise when the stress hormones are released. Never attempt this without first discussing it thoroughly with your physician/health care team, and use this approach only after extensive testing has demonstrated that the extra insulin is really needed. For most short, strenuous events, it may be just as easy to correct any high blood sugars that may occur after the event is completed.

How Exercise Intensity And Duration Impact Your Blood Sugar

Mild Versus Strenuous Exercise

At rest, free fatty acids supply most of our fuel. During mild exercise, like walking or golfing, energy is still largely obtained from fats rather than sugar, and for this reason, a drop in the blood sugar is less likely than in more strenuous exercise.

Whether you walk or run a mile makes no difference in the amount of energy you use. Moving yourself an identical distance at any speed uses the same number of calories. However, the source of the calories used will depend on the intensity of the activity. In a one-mile walk, only 20 percent of the calories come from glucose. A satisfying 80 percent of the calories come from fat.

Unlike walking, running one mile at a strenuous pace can burn as much as 80 percent of your calories from glucose. As exercise intensity increases, so too does the amount of glucose that is needed as fuel. Because more carbohydrate is used during intense exercise, the blood sugar is also more likely to drop. Strenuous exercise, therefore, has to be balanced with more carbohydrate intake or a larger reduction in insulin than mild exercise (except in the case of very strenuous anaerobic exercise as noted above).

Anaerobic Exercise

One way of categorizing exercise is the "talk test". As long as you can talk during exercise, it is aerobic exercise. If you cannot carry on a conversation while exercising, your effort has risen into the anaerobic ("without oxygen") range. Jogging, bike riding, even fast walking can become anaerobic if done to excess. Examples of pure anaerobic exercise are the 100-yard dash and power weight lifting.

During short periods of anaerobic exercise, the blood sugar can rise despite seemingly adequate insulin levels because glucose is mobilized very rapidly from glycogen stores to supply fuel. This can overwhelm the current insulin level and cause the blood sugar to go up. If experience shows that your blood sugar rises after this type of exercise, check with your physician for more specific instructions on insulin adjustments.

Duration

The length of exercise also influences how much carbohydrate is used. Activities that last longer are more likely to drop your blood sugar. For instance, a 30- minute walk might not affect the blood sugar, but walking for 60 minutes may require extra carbohydrate or a reduced carb bolus.

Any time exercise lasts longer than 40 to 60 minutes, the body has to switch from using its limited stores of glucose and glycogen to using its very large stores of fat as fuel. In an example of a normal person over several hours, the person is getting 80 percent of the needed energy from glucose at the start of fairly strenuous exercise. After three hours, an equal amount of energy is coming from glucose and fat. By the end of six hours of exercise, these fuels have switched priority, and almost 80 percent of the energy is coming from fat.

Remember, though, this person has a normal pancreas that automatically lowers insulin levels. If someone with diabetes does not reduce insulin doses for this same exercise, it will be hard to access body fat for fuel. Instead, they will have to eat carbohydrate to supply this energy.

In the normal person, the total energy used in six hours of exercise is 3,347 calories. Half of this person's

What Is Training?

The American College of Sports medicine says you are training when you exercise:

• Three to five times a week

• For 15 to 60 minutes at a time

• At 60% to 90% of your maximum heart rate (220 minus your age)

• While using any large muscle mass

Caution: if you have autonomic neuropathy, your heart rate will NOT be accurate for training. Discuss with your physician.

calories comes from carbohydrate and half from fat. For exercisers with diabetes, if they did not reduce their insulin level during this six-hour exercise, the excess insulin would blunt access to internal fat and glycogen stores. Most of the 3,347 calories used would have to be eaten as carbohydrate to keep the blood sugar from falling. This is equivalent to eating almost two pounds of pure sugar, or drinking twenty 12-ounce cans of regular soda. Obviously, lowering insulin levels during long periods of exercise is required to prevent both low blood sugars and stomach aches.

Experience can help you improve your estimates of how the length and intensity of upcoming activities is balanced with extra carbohydrate or less insulin. The concept of ExCarbs introduced in the next chapter will provide better tools to do this.

How To Prevent Insulin Reactions

When low blood sugars occur during or just after exercise or work, symptoms may be difficult to recognize. Symptoms like sweating and shaking can be caused by either exercise or a low blood sugar. Other warning signs may go unnoticed because you are focusing on the activity. To avoid low blood sugars during exercise and at the same time improve performance, frequent blood sugar monitoring is recommended.

Frequent testing also can prevent or quickly catch any delayed insulin reactions that might occur hours after strenuous exercise. These reactions can occur up to 36 hours after strenuous or prolonged exercise or work, and they often happen during the night following the activity. Delayed reactions are caused by a drop in blood sugar as the muscles and liver gradually remove sugar from the blood to replenish their glycogen stores depleted by the day's exercise. To avoid delayed reactions, test often, reduce basal rates, and eat extra carbohydrate not covered with a bolus, especially at bedtime.

During exercise, having a supply of quick-acting, high-carbohydrate snacks helps prevent and/or treat insulin reactions. Be especially careful during and after occasional, intense exercise for which you are not trained. Canoe trips, backpacking, skiing, horseback riding, spring cleaning, home remodeling, heavy work in the garden or even washing the car can all create an unusually fast drop in the blood sugar because you do not do these activities every day.

Someone who is poorly trained may need to offset unusually strenuous activities like these with a greater reduction in their basals and boluses to avoid low blood sugars. Since people vary, let your personal experience with the same or similar activity can guide your adjustments. Good record keeping is especially helpful for handling activities in which you participate only occasionally and also for periods of training.

A normal blood sugar during and after exercise indicates that an ideal balance has been reached between insulin doses, carbohydrate intake, and the use of glucose and fat as fuels.

Beginning "New" Exercise

Any new exercise will cause your muscle cells to move more glucose into glycogen stores in preparation for similar exercise in the future. Because this extra glucose is required, the risk of a low blood sugar increases following any exercise that you have not participated in within the last three to five days. These lows often occur during sleep that night. As training improves and glycogen stores become enlarged, muscle efficiency increases and blood sugars become less likely to drop.

The Value Of Blood Sugar Trending

The information most professional athletes with diabetes want to know is the trend line for their blood sugars prior to, during, and after events. They want to know where their blood sugars are, but also in which direction they are heading and how fast.

Athletes like Jay Leeuwenburg, offensive lineman for the Cincinnati Bengals, will test his blood sugars every 20 to 30 minutes for about two hours before a football game begins, during the game as often as possible, and again for the same period after the game. His frequent testing allows him to pick up trends in his blood sugars and correct as needed with carbohydrates or insulin to keep his blood sugars close to normal. The postgame readings help him avoid unexpected highs and lows after his very strenuous exercise.

Trending will, of course, become much easier as continuous blood sugar monitors become more widely available. Continuous monitors let you quickly determine the direction of your blood sugars.

A drop in the blood sugar also is more likely when an exercise involves a new muscle group. For example, a runner who begins to bike will experience a larger blood sugar drop after biking than after running, even if the energy used for each exercise is the same. This extra drop is caused by the formation of new glycogen stores in the relatively untrained leg muscles required for biking but not for running.

Advantage Of Physical Training

When you do structured exercise regularly, not only do you tone up and slim down, but blood sugar fluctuations can also be reduced. The reason physical training makes such a difference is that training builds glycogen stores. This glycogen, stored in liver and muscle cells, acts as a large account that can be drawn upon to keep your glucose funds from running low.

During exercise, someone who is in shape will use 25 percent less glucose than someone who is not trained. The fit individual stores more glycogen internally in his or her muscles and uses these glycogen stores more efficiently. This, added to reduced basals and boluses, means the fit person needs less carbohydrate in snacks or supplements to prevent insulin reactions. Blood sugar control is much easier when you are trained.

Exercise is an important ingredient in anyone's health program, especially someone who has diabetes. With planning, blood sugar monitoring, and adjusting carbs and insulin, you can exercise with a renewed spirit of fun, enjoyment, and confidence.

Example: Mountain Climber Colby Smith

A good example of the benefits of training can be seen in Colby Smith, a member of the International Diabetes Athletes Association. Colby climbs mountains, not just any mountain but the highest mountain on each of the seven continents. Although his diabetes makes this more challenging, he has climbed three of the seven highest mountains already, going up to almost 23,000 feet.

Up to about 14,000 feet, he tests with a Chemstrip, a visual strip on which he places a drop of blood and holds in his mouth to keep it warm as the reading is processed. Then he compares the strip visually to a color grid on the can to get his reading. Blood sugar testing becomes practically impossible above 14,000 to 16,000 feet due to extreme cold, wind, and low oxygen levels. What allows Colby to maintain good control without blood sugar testing is the remarkably stable blood sugars he has while climbing. Colby's blood sugars typically range between 70 and 80 mg/dl (3.9 and 4.4 mmol) on climbs! Much of the reason for his excellent control is that he has built massive glycogen stores during his previous training. Like diabetic shock absorbers, his muscle and glycogen stores soak up excess glucose from the bloodstream and release it as needed.

ExCarbs For Exercise

People with diabetes often avoid exercise. They may want to exercise because it's fun, makes them feel better, and improves their health. But what happens? A long walk, some rollerblading, or painting the house, and their blood sugar drops. Then a hastily eaten candy bar sends the blood sugar soaring. Some extra insulin corrects the high but then the blood sugar goes low again.

Or perhaps after exercising for a half hour in the morning, the blood sugar rises rather than falls as expected, and it takes the rest of the day to regain control. Maybe a frightening nighttime low follows the exercise of the day. No wonder exercise loses it appeal after such experiences.

To avoid control problems related to exercise, it's critical to know how to make adjustments in your carbohydrate intake, basals, and boluses. One way to quantify the impact an exercise event will have is to calculate what is called ExCarbs.

This chapter discusses

- What ExCarbs are
- How to use ExCarbs to control blood sugars during exercise
- How to lower basals and boluses with ExCarbs

What Are ExCarbs?

Although exact exercise rules are not possible, ExCarbs provide a yardstick to measure how a particular aerobic exercise affects your blood sugar. (Do not use ExCarbs with anaerobic exercise. Anaerobic exercise often drives the blood sugar up.) Exercise physiologists have long known how many calories are consumed in different activities. They also know what percentage of these calories need to come from carbohydrate. ExCarbs uses this information about carbs burned in specific types of exercise to help you stay in control during exercise.

ExCarbs allow you to balance exercise

1. By eating more carbohydrate (easy to do and good for maintaining your current weight)
2. By lowering insulin doses (great for weight loss)
3. Using a combination of the two (flexible, customized to your needs)

More Carbohydrate

An easy way to keep blood sugars normal while exercising is to eat the exact amount of carbohydrate that is burned during the exercise you are engaged in. Simply look up your planned exercise in Table 19.1 and determine how many carbohydrates you need for this exercise. Then eat foods with this number of grams of carbohydrate during and after the exercise to maintain control.

This table has been set up for body weights of 100 lbs., 150 lbs., and 200 lbs. and for different intensity levels of exercise. If you weigh 150 pounds and walk 3 miles in an hour, using the table you see that you use 22 grams of carbs. This is equal to an average-sized apple or a cup of milk plus a graham cracker. If you walk at the same pace for two hours rather than one, you'll need 44 grams of carbohydrate, while if you walk for only 30 minutes, you will need 11 grams.

If instead of walking, you run the same 3 miles at a speed of 8 m.p.h., you'll need 53 grams of carbohydrate, even though the run lasts only 22 minutes (145 grams times 22 min. ÷ 60 min.). This is more than twice the amount needed for the leisurely one-hour walk over the same ground!

The numbers listed in the table are usually the maximum amount of carbs needed for each hour of exercise to prevent a low blood sugar. Usually, a full replacement of these carbohydrates is not necessary right at the time of exercise. Over a 10- to 36-hour period following the exercise, most or all of these carbohydrates will have to be replaced or balanced with basal and bolus reductions. The full carb replacement may be needed at the time of the exercise if excess amounts of insulin are present in the blood. Here the excess insulin blocks access to internal glycogen and fat stores and makes eating the only way to deliver fuel to the exercising muscles.

Table 19.1 ExCarbs: Grams Of Carb Used Per Hour For Various Activities

Activity	Weight 100 lbs.	Weight 150 lbs.	Weight 200 lbs.	% calories from carbs	Activity	Weight 100 lbs.	Weight 150 lbs.	Weight 200 lbs.	% calories from carbs
baseball	25	38	50	40%	running				
basketball					5 mph	45	68	90	50%
moderate	35				8 mph	96	145	190	65%
vigorous	59				10 mph	126	189	252	70%
bicycling					shovelling	31	45	57	50%
6 mph	20	27	34	40%	skating				
10 mph	35	48	61	50%	moderate	25	34	43	40%
14 mph	60	83	105	60%	vigorous	67	92	117	60%
18 mph	95	130	165	65%	skiing				
20 mph	122	168	214	70%	crosscntry 5 mph	76	105	133	60%
dancing					downhill	52	72	92	50%
moderate	17	25	33	40%	water	42	58	74	50%
vigorous	28	43	57	50%	soccer	45	67	89	50%
digging	45	65	83	50%	swimming				
eating	6	8	10	30%	slow crawl	41	56	71	50%
golf (pullcart)	23	35	46	40%	fast crawl	69	95	121	60%
handball	59	88	117	60%	tennis				
jump rope 80/min	73	109	145	65%	moderate	28	41	55	40%
mopping	16	23	30	30%	vigorous	59	88	117	60%
mountain climbing	60	90	120	60%	volleyball				
outside painting	21	31	42	40%	moderate	23	34	45	40%
raking leaves	19	28	38	30%	vigorous	59	88	117	60%
					walking				
					3 mph	15	22	29	30%
					4.5 mph	30	45	59	45%

Replacing the carbohydrate used as fuel during exercise requires that you know how to count carbohydrates. To review how to count carbohydrates, see Chapter 7.

Less Insulin

As exercise increases in length and intensity, reducing insulin doses becomes more and more necessary. Long, intense periods of exercise require that basals and boluses be reduced before exercise and may require that doses remain reduced for as long as 36 hours afterward. Whether boluses or basals are reduced depends on the length of the exercise, the timing in relation to the previous meal bolus, and of course whether the exercise was planned. Keep in mind that with any insulin reduction on the pump there will always be a time lag between the reduction time and when the level of insulin in the blood actually begins to drop.

Reducing Humalog meal boluses is ideal for moderate or strenuous exercise that will begin within 90 minutes after eating. For strenuous exercise that will last 60 minutes or more and moderate exercise over 90 minutes, a reduction in the basal rate should be considered also. Remember that once a basal rate has been lowered, it will take another 60 to 90 minutes with Humalog insulin, or 90 to 120 minutes with Regular insulin, before the insulin level in the blood actually begins to drop. Therefore, basal reductions have to be started at least one to three hours before exercise begins.

For instance, exercise that starts an hour after breakfast and that lasts more than 90 minutes may require a reduction in the breakfast bolus, along with a reduction in the morning and afternoon basal rates. Table 19.2 provides a timetable to show the time lapse after various types of insulin are lowered before an actual drop in the blood insulin level will begin.

One benefit of reducing insulin levels is that it allows a greater release of fuel from internal stores of glycogen and fat so that eating additional food is not as necessary. This helps those who want to lose weight and also those who participate in long periods of activity but don't want to consume the large portions of carbohydrate that would otherwise be required.

When reducing basals and boluses for exercise, keep in mind your current level of training, the duration and intensity of exercise, and whether your current insulin doses are correctly set. (Normal blood sugars most of the time are a good sign of correct insulin doses.)

Your level of training can make a tremendous difference in the need to adjust insulin. When you perform an exercise you rarely engage in, you are likely to need greater basal and bolus reductions than for a equivalent amount of exercise that is routine. Before starting an exercise training program, some reduction in boluses and basal rates likely will be needed. People who exercise regularly and are in good control already have lowered their insulin doses to compensate, so little to no adjustment of the insulin dose is needed for a regular session of exercise.

Use Your Insulin-To-Carb Ratio To Reduce Insulin For Exercise

ExCarbs also can act as a guide for reducing insulin doses. You only need to know your insulin-to-carbohydrate ratio, provided in Table 10.1 (p. 92). The rules used in these tables say that the number of grams of carbohydrate covered by one unit of Humalog can be approximated by dividing 500 by your TDD in Table 11.1 (p. 107).

For instance, someone with Type 1 diabetes who requires 30 total units of insulin each day and uses half the TDD as basal will need about one unit of Humalog for every 17 grams of carbohydrate (500 divided by 30 equals 16.7), while someone else who uses 50 units a day will need about one unit of Humalog for each ten grams of carbohydrate (500 divided by 50 equals 10).

Let's try using the 500 Rule to lower Humalog doses for exercise. We'll calculate an insulin dose reduction for someone who weighs 150 pounds and uses 38 units of insulin a day with 50% basal. Dividing the daily average insulin dose of 38 units into 500, we get 13, which means this person needs approximately one unit of Humalog for every 13 grams of carbohydrate. We are assuming the person has good control on insulin pump therapy.

> ### International Diabetes Athletes Association
>
> The IDAA is a great place to meet other active people with diabetes. A terrific three day North American Conference is held each year with talks and workshops by diabetes specialists involved in a wide variety of sports.
>
> A finding presented by exercise specialists and confirmed by participants is that the more body mass one has, the easier blood sugar control becomes. This suggests that a combination of aerobic exercise for cardiovascular fitness plus strength training for muscle mass is important in diabetes.
>
> Contact IDAA at 1647-B West Bethany Home Road; Phoenix, AZ 85015; info: (602) 433-2113, membership: (800) 898-4311, or visit www.diabetes-exercise.org

Now look at Table 19.1. For this 150-pound person, a 30-minute run at 8 m.p.h. translates into at most 72 grams of ExCarbs (145 grams per hour times a half hour). Knowing this, we can easily figure that the run will be equivalent to 72 grams of carb divided by 13 grams per unit of insulin, or a total of five to six units of Humalog (72/13 = 5.5).

Our runner may then choose to eat extra carbohydrates, lower a meal bolus, or both. (A basal reduction won't be needed for a run that lasts only a half hour.) Using only carb replacement, he/she would eat as many as 72 extra grams of carbohydrate not covered with any carb boluses. These carbohydrates help meet the extra demand for energy that the run requires. A good way to replace the ExCarbs is to have about a third of the carbs before the run and to eat the other two-thirds over several hours later in the day.

Using only an insulin reduction, our runner can reduce the meal bolus. Let's say the run will occur an hour after eating. Calculating the number of carbs in the meal, these can be covered with five (5 u x 13 gr/u = 65 grams equivalent) to

> ## Lows, Highs and Exercise
>
> • The longer and more strenuous an exercise or activity, the more likely the blood sugar will go low and the greater the need to lower your insulin doses.
>
> • The less trained you are for an activity, the more likely your blood sugar will go low and the greater the need to lower insulin doses.
>
> • Strenuous or anaerobic exercise may raise the blood sugar if glucose is mobilized faster than it can be moved into cells by the prevailing insulin level.

six (6 u x 13 gr/u = 78 grams equivalent) fewer units of insulin than ordinarily used.

More Carbs And Less Insulin

A combination of extra carbohydrates plus a reduction in boluses and basal rates, usually provides the best control for all but short periods of exercise. For example, our 30-minute runner could reduce the meal bolus by three units, and eat up to 36 grams of extra carbohydrate that day.

Recommendations for making carbohydrate and basal/bolus adjustments based on duration and intensity of exercise are given in Table 19.2 on page 177. Both the intensity and the duration of exercise affect how it can be balanced with eating extra carbs or reducing basals and boluses. Basically, the longer and more strenuous the exercise, the greater the adjustment required, and the more likely that basals and/or boluses will need to be lowered.

The length of exercise is easy to determine with a watch or clock, but intensity is a different matter. Intensity is highly specific to each individual. Two people may be running side by side at the same speed, but one may be running at maximum intensity, while for the other, the same exercise may be mild.

In Table 19.2, mild exercise is any extra activity that is relatively easy for you to do, such as casual walking. Moderate exercise involves something that makes you breathe harder but which you could do for some time, such as brisk walking or jogging. Intense exercise involves anything that causes deep breathing but still allows you to carry on a conversation. Examples are race walking or a steady, fast bike ride. All of these are aerobic exercises.

Adjustments of insulin and carbohydrate vary greatly from individual to individual. The reasons for these variations are complex and not completely understood. Some people may need to lower their boluses and basals only slightly for exercise; others may find that a large insulin reduction is the only way to control their blood sugars. For some, the breakfast bolus does not need to be lowered for morning exercise, but when they do the same exercise later in the day, they have to reduce their lunch or dinner bolus. The only way to determine your own response is to experiment, record your results, and discuss these with your physician/health care team.

How To Lower High Blood Sugars With Exercise

There is also a third way to balance exercise. Exercise can be used to bring down high blood sugars. If your blood sugar is high before you exercise, the exercise can be used to lower the high reading instead of taking a high blood sugar bolus.

Let's say you weigh 200 pounds, use 50 units of insulin a day (50 percent basal), and generally have good control. From Table 10.1 (p. 92) you'll need one unit of Humalog for each 10 grams of carbohydrate and one unit of Humalog for each 36 points you wish to lower your blood sugar. You wake up one morning with a blood sugar of 172. You want to eat 100 grams of carbohydrate for breakfast and then ride a bike at 14 m.p.h. for one hour. If you weren't planning to ride, you would take 10 units of Humalog for your breakfast carbohydrate, plus an extra 2 units of Humalog for the high blood sugar (72/36 = 2.0).

From Table 19.1 you calculate that weighing 200 pounds and riding 14 m.p.h. for an hour, you'll need the equivalent of 105 grams of ExCarbs for the ride.

These 105 grams can be translated into these choices:
- An extra 105 grams of "free" carbohydrate during the day
- 10.5 fewer units of Humalog (105 grams ÷ 10 grams per unit)
- A blood sugar drop of 378 points (36 per unit of Humalog X 10.5 units)
- Some combination of the above

Two of many possible choices:

1. Take your normal bolus of insulin—10 Humalog for breakfast, plus the 2 extra units to lower the high blood sugar. Then eat 100 grams of carbohydrate for breakfast, plus another 105 grams of free carbohydrate during and after the bike ride. (The extra carbohydrate equals seven average slices of bread.)

2. Take six units of Humalog to cover breakfast (50 percent of the usual breakfast bolus) and 1 unit to lower the blood sugar. This is 5 units less insulin, or 5 times 10 grams per unit equals 50 grams of carbs. Then eat your usual 100 grams of carbohydrate for breakfast. Only 65 grams of free carbohydrate (105 extra grams required for the ride, minus the 50 grams that were not covered by insulin) will then be needed during and after the ride. (Free carbohydrate means carb not covered by a bolus.)

How Far Can Insulin Doses Be Reduced For Exercise?

A major consideration in calculating basal and bolus reductions for exercise is that there are limits to how far insulin doses can be reduced. Let's say your current insulin dose is correct (i.e., your control is quite good). You start a strenuous running program in preparation for a marathon. With multi-mile runs on your training days, you find you use enough ExCarbs that it seems possible to skip your entire insulin dose.

Can all your insulin really be eliminated if you exercise long enough? With Type 2 diabetes, this can be done occasionally with planning if residual insulin production is adequate. With Type 1 diabetes, however, no internal insulin production occurs, and therefore, basal and bolus insulin can never be eliminated totally.

For an explanation of this, let's look at marathon runners who do not have diabetes. Even during maximum training, a marathoner's blood insulin level will drop no further than to about half of its original level. This tells us that in Type 1 diabetes, total insulin intake should be reduced by no more than 40 to 50 percent from the original dose for even the most intense exercise programs.

So keep in mind that, unlike carbohydrates which can be added as needed, insulin doses can be reduced only so far. Your TDD cannot be reduced more than 40 to 50 percent, unless you are also losing weight or your original insulin doses were too high.

This limit is created by

1. The need to cover meal carbohydrates with enough insulin to keep the blood sugar from rising at the time the meal is eaten.

2. The need for sufficient background insulin to allow glucose to enter cells and to keep the massive internal stores of glucose and fat from being released.

3. The need to prevent ketoacidosis, which results whenever there is a marked reduction of insulin doses.

Of course, never take any dose of insulin that seems inappropriate. If you usually take three units of Humalog for your meal prior to the start of your exercise and your blood sugar control has been great, do not take more or less than this amount, even if a different dose is suggested by the ExCarb system, the 500 Rule, or any other rule. Your own blood sugars are always your best guide. Check with your physician before using ExCarbs as a system for reducing insulin and increasing carbohydrates.

When To Eat Your Carbs

The ExCarb table shows how many total carbs are required, but you also need to know when to eat them. Even if your blood sugar is normal before exercise, all this carbohydrate does not need to be eaten right away.

For example, during the first 30 minutes of moderately strenuous exercise, like running at 6 m.p.h., about half the fuel is derived from carbs. Of this carbohydrate, most comes directly from internal glycogen stores in the leg muscles. Only about 10 percent comes directly out of the blood as glucose. Only this blood-derived glucose has to be immediately replaced through eating or from the production and release of glucose by the liver. Even if your insulin levels are high during a 30-minute run, only

16 percent of the calories come directly from the blood as glucose. This means that the glucose removed from glycogen stores can, in most instances, be replaced after the exercise is finished, unless your experience tells you otherwise.

In the first 30 minutes of exercise, local muscle glycogen contributes about five times as much glucose as the blood does. As the run continues beyond 30 minutes, more and more glucose begins to be drawn from the bloodstream. The amount of glucose needed from the blood climbs gradually during the first couple of hours to about 40 percent. This is why eating or drinking carbohydrate becomes more necessary and why the blood sugar becomes more likely to drop as exercise continues.

The insulin level drops about 50 percent for the nondiabetic during the first hour or two of moderate exercise. In diabetes, if insulin levels do not drop during this time, more food is required to keep the blood sugar from falling. Eating is always the major way to supply fuel when insulin levels are set too high.

Most of the carbohydrate burned for exercise that lasts only 30 to 45 minutes comes from internal glycogen stores rather than the blood. If insulin levels are correctly lowered when exercise starts, these internal glycogen stores can release their stored glucose as fuel for the exercise.

The longer and more intense the exercise, the longer it takes to rebuild muscle glycogen stores afterwards. After intense exercise the blood sugar may drop for periods up to 36 hours as glucose is gradually removed from the bloodstream and used to rebuild glycogen stores. As mentioned earlier, this means that not all of the carbohydrate used

Table 19.2 Carb, Bolus, and Basal Adjustments To Balance Exercise For 100 lb. Person

Exercise Duration	Exercise Intensity								
	Mild			Moderate			Intense		
	Excarbs*	Bolus	Basal	Excarbs*	Bolus	Basal	Excarbs*	Bolus	Basal
15 min	+0 g	normal	normal	+0 g	normal	normal	+20 g	-10%	normal
30 min	+10 g	normal	normal	+20 g	-10%	normal	+40 g	-20%	normal
45 min	+18 g	-10%	normal	+30 g	-20%	normal	+50 g	-30%	normal
60 min	+25 g	-15%	normal	+40 g	-30%	normal	+60 g	-40%	-10%
90 min	+38 g	-20%	normal	+55 g	-45%	-20%	+90 g	-50%	-20%
120 mn	+50 g	-30%	normal	+70 g	-60%	-20%	+110 g	-70%	-30%
240 min	+80 g	-50%	- 10%	+120 g	-60%	-20%	+200 g	-70%	-40%

These are estimates only; they must be individually adjusted through testing.
*Important: Excarb values above are for an 100 lb. person. They must be adjusted for your weight and level of training. At 200 lbs, you will need TWICE the carbohydrate. If untrained, you may need more carbs; if trained, you may need less than these amounts.

in exercise has to be eaten immediately. Most athletes with diabetes add carbs to their bedtime snack to prevent a nighttime drop. Depending on its length and intensity, your exercise may require you to eat carbs before, during, and up to 36 hours after it.

Wise Exercise

Keep in mind your previous experiences with similar exercise. Also, be sure your insulin doses and carbohydrate intake are matched to your normal daily lifestyle before attempting to make adjustments for exercise.

Discuss your exercise program with your physician/health care team, monitor your blood sugars often, and use all the information and tips on exercise provided in this book.

Test your blood sugar often when exercising, or use a continuous monitoring device. This feedback lets you adjust your insulin doses more precisely to the length and intensity of your exercise. For rapid correction of low blood sugars during exercise, carry some fast-acting carbohydrates, like glucose tablets or SweetTarts.™ To stay hydrated and to bring down a high blood sugar, always carry water or other noncaloric fluids.

If you plan to participate in a strenuous activity like a triathelon, marathon, century, etc., tap the experience of other athletes with diabetes who have encountered these challenges before you. You can usually get a quick referral to another athlete who participates in your sport through the International Diabetes Athletes Association at (602) 433-2113. Discuss your findings with your physician.

Exercise can make you feel and look younger and can increase your sense of well-being, especially if you learn how to master your blood sugar control in the process. Exercise also appears to be an important way to reduce the risk of complications and to live a long, healthy life.

When ExCarbs Don't Work

What if the ExCarb system doesn't work? Don't feel bad! There are lots of competing factors, listed in Chapter 18, that can influence the blood sugar during exercise. Consider the following factors that can affect your exercise:

Incorrect Insulin Doses

A key question to ask if the ExCarb system is not working is, "Are my current basals and boluses set properly?"

As an example of someone who has these insulin doses set too high, consider a person who has frequent low blood sugars in the afternoon but who decides to start exercising at 3 p.m. without first lowering the afternoon basal or lunch bolus, or eating extra ExCarbs. The insulin reaction that follows will now be quite severe but should not be blamed on the exercise. Blame it instead on the underlying problem--excess insulin and inadequate carbs at the time chosen for exercise.

As an example of someone with insulin doses set too low, consider a person who wakes up in the morning with a reading of 180 mg/dl (10 mmol) because her early morning basal is set too low and then goes jogging for 30 minutes. She is surprised when her blood sugar rises to 240 mg/dl (13.3 mmol) on her return. Again, the exercise is not to blame. The cause is the underlying lack of insulin that allows the glycogen stores in the liver and muscles to be released into the blood easily. and can't help this released glucose move into the muscles for use as fuel. Her blood sugar control could have been improved by taking a small dose of Humalog before starting to jog, or, even better, by maintaining blood sugar control during the previous night by raising the nighttime basal rates.

Stress Hormones

A less predicable factor is the effect of stress hormones. Large amounts of stress hormones are often released at the start of a competitive event, like a swim meet, a 10K run, or a century bike ride. Nervousness at the starting line is a sign of stress hormones at work. Blood sugars often rise unexpectedly in these circumstances. You might want to take extra insulin very carefully (seek advise of your doctor) to cover this rise and lower the high blood sugar for shorter events like a 10K. You probably won't need to lower it for a century bike ride; the exercise itself in longer events lowers the high.

Unusual Circumstances

Problems can also creep in when exercise conditions change. If you usually walk two miles on flat ground but decide to walk the same distance in hilly country, you'll use more fuel climbing these grades. A strong headwind can increase carbohydrate consumption by about one percent for each extra mile per hour of headwind (i.e., for a 10 m.p.h. headwind, increase carbs by 10 percent). Walking in dry sand or soft snow can double the amount of carbohydrate needed for the same walk on firm ground.

Activities that have uneven pacing, like spring cleaning or playing football, can also cause problems. It's hard to predict whether you'll spend the next hour sorting through the closet for throwaways or moving furniture. Maybe you'll sit on the bench during the entire game or maybe you'll be giving your all on the field. Luckily, most activities don't suffer from this much unpredictability.

Exercise Tips

• Test blood sugars more often while exercising and in the following 24 to 36 hours. Wear a continuous blood sugar monitor, if possible, and set the low blood sugar warning alarm.

• Lower your basals and boluses before long periods of exercise or activity for better access to internal stores of glucose and fat. (Also helps prevent low blood sugars.)

• For performance and safety, keep the blood sugar between 70 and 150 mg/dl (3.9 to 8.3 mmol) during exercise, and try to keep it from dropping below 65 mg/dl afterward.

• Normal meal boluses may need to be lowered by 50 percent or more when taken before or during vigorous exercise or heavy work. For example, if one unit is normally taken for each 10 grams of carbohydrate, try taking only one unit for every 20 grams when working or exercising hard. Some vigorous exercise may require the total elimination of a bolus for the carbohydrate in a meal.

• A bolus taken to bring down high blood sugars may also need to be lowered by 50 percent or more when given before or during longer periods of moderate or strenuous exercise.

• For intense activities that last a day or two, such as a weekend backpacking trip, try lowering the basal dose by 20 percent to 40 percent and the meal bolus by 50 percent. Lower the basal insulin 60 to 90 minutes ahead of the activity for Humalog insulin and 90 to 120 minutes for Regular. Keep the basal rates somewhat lower than normal for about 24 to 36 hours following the exercise.

• The basal insulin rate rarely needs to be lowered for short, random periods of exercise, but it may need to be reduced gradually if your overall physical fitness improves.

• Remember, never lower your TDD more than 50 percent for even the most strenuous exercise.

• Before making any changes in your own insulin doses, discuss these suggestions with your physician. They may not be appropriate for you.

An excellent diet cannot make an average athlete great,
but a poor diet can make a great athlete average.

Children and Teens

by Barb Schreiner, R.N., M.N., C.D.E., and Shannon Brow, R.N., B.S., C.D.E. of Texas Children's Hospital, Houston, TX

Although insulin pumps and pump therapy have been around for over two decades, using pumps with children and teens has just begun to gain acceptance. There are several reasons a pump can be an ideal tool for the child or teen with diabetes. The precise size and timing of insulin doses is ideal for children and teens, who are often very sensitive to insulin and need small doses. The Dawn Phenomenon is common, requiring a precise dose increase at an exact time during the night. Pumps handle this need for precision dosing much better than do injections of long-acting and fast-acting insulin.

To gain all the benefits of this excellent tool, pump therapy in children and teens requires a few special considerations. Determining which child or teen will do well on the pump, specific techniques for using the pump, and tips about specific pump programming for young pumpers all will be discussed in this chapter.

Why Pump? Myths And Half-Truths

Why do kids, teens, parents, and diabetes professionals choose to use the pump? The reasons can be quite varied. Kids will often consider a pump because, "I can eat whatever and whenever I want!" They'll say "I don't have to take extra shots anymore!" They may mistakenly believe they also can quit fingerstick blood sugar testing because "the pump will know what my sugar is and how much insulin to give."

Parents will choose pumps for their children to "simplify diabetes." The flexibility in daily schedules, in handling sick days, and in keeping up with the child's or teen's growth spurts seem wonderful to parents.; the parents feel "it will control the blood sugar better," because they recognize that the pump affords a precision that no other insulin delivery system can provide. After using the pump for a while, some parents even gain "peace of mind." They notice that the pump and its benefits have made them less anxious about their children. They "hover" less, worry less, and regain their confidence as parents.

Diabetes professionals look to the pump for children and teens to delay or prevent diabetes complications, to prevent repeated hospitalizations, to decrease episodes of severe hypoglycemia, and to help control blood glucose during the Dawn Phenomenon or during growth spurts.

People's reasons for pumping are sometimes in conflict or unrealistic. When thinking about pump therapy, it is important for you as a parent, child, or teen to share your reasons for wanting a pump with your diabetes team. In return, your diabetes team will want to be sure that a pump is the best choice for you.

How can you know when a child or teen is ready for a pump? There are several factors about young potential pumpers to consider:

- Maturity
- Problem-solving ability
- Responsibility, such as remembering to give boluses
- Vigorous activity

The key to successful pump therapy in children and teens is that the person who will wear the pump has to want to wear it! If there is no "buy in" from the child or teen, the therapy may be doomed to fail. Because children and teens often want to please their parents and their diabetes team, they may agree to pump therapy because Mom and Dad desperately want it. They then may feel trapped and begin to sabotage the program as a way out.

When unclear expectations can backfire

Jenny was rather lukewarm about pumps. She really didn't want a needle or catheter always in her skin. She worried about always being connected to a "machine," but her mom and dad were insistent. They were convinced that a pump would provide perfect blood sugar control and that would keep Jenny safe from complications.

Jenny finally agreed to start pump therapy, but she had difficulty inserting the infusion sets time after time. She complained of frequent alarms, and would forget to take her boluses. Jenny was telling her parents and health care team indirectly in these ways that pump therapy was not right for her at this time. She confided to her nurse that she couldn't find a way to tell her mom and dad that she didn't want to do it anymore. After all, they had confidence in the approach, they had invested time and money, and they were looking out for her best interests. Jenny's diabetes team worked with the family to find a different insulin program to follow until she was ready to commit to pump therapy. Jenny discontinued the pump until she had time to mature and the family had time to clarify their goals. Two years later, she returned to pump therapy and was much more successful!

As a parent, be realistic about what pump therapy can do. Here are some common myths:

Myth: My child or teen will have perfect blood sugar control once on the pump.

Truth: Blood sugar control probably will improve, but no one's control is perfect.

Myth: The pump will prevent all complications.

Truth: The good control of blood sugars possible on the pump decreases the risk of complications greatly. However, some complications may still occur.

Myth: Pump therapy will be easier and will take less time.

Truth: Pump therapy becomes easier as you do it, but learning the techniques is arduous and time-consuming. Changing the infusion site, which is necessary at least every three days, will continue to take more time than an injection.

Myth: My child or teen won't have to monitor as much.

Truth: The need to monitor will never decrease. At first, as you are testing basals and boluses, the number of blood sugar tests required will increase. After that, you will need to test before each meal and at bedtime and any other time you are unsure about your blood sugar level.

One of our physician friends and a pump wearer, Dr. Stephen W. Ponder, frequently talks with families about pump therapy. He uses this analogy: Think about the pump like your family dog on a leash. Imagine bringing your dog on the leash along as you take a bath, eat out at restaurants, or when you play your championship soccer game. Imagine sleeping with your dog on a leash in your bed! Imagine taking the leashed dog to school, being around your friends, and taking him on a date with you. If you think you can do this for three days, you probably have an idea what it would be like to have an insulin pump connected to your body 24 hours a day, 7 days a week!

Here are three youngsters who are considering pump therapy. Notice how different their needs and concerns are.

Sally

Sally is 12 and has been using an intensive insulin management program for several months. She is skilled at making insulin dose decisions and recently had a HbA1c of 7.1 % with a normal of 6% or less at the lab she uses. She is very involved with school activities and athletics and has a schedule that varies widely from day to day. Sally heard about pump therapy at diabetes camp this summer, and decided she wanted to try it. Sally's goals for pump therapy include more flexibility in daily routine and taking fewer injections, and her parents support her decision.

Is Sally a good candidate for pump therapy?

Ralph

At age 15 Ralph has had several difficult years managing his diabetes. He has been hospitalized twice for DKA in the past year. Although he tests frequently, he does not interpret the results nor use them to make dose adjustments. His last HbA1c was 9.2%. Ralph is mostly in charge of his diabetes care. He admits to missing doses of insulin occasionally, mainly because it is too inconvenient to carry his insulin with him. He wants to try something different. During his last hospitalization, Ralph explained the reason he went into DKA. While spending the weekend with a friend, he dropped his bottle of insulin and was too embarrassed to ask the friend's parents to help him obtain more insulin. He decided to just watch what he ate that weekend. He wants to play sports, and he knows he can't afford to miss any more school.

Is Ralph a good candidate for pump therapy?

Lauren

Lauren is an 8-year-old who has had several recent episodes of severe hypoglycemia. These have occurred despite creative and individualized insulin programs, frequent blood glucose monitoring and dose adjustments, and close cooperation between parents and the diabetes team. Her last HbA1c was 7.8 %. Her daily schedule varies, with swimming on some days, dance on others, and no activity on other days. Her diabetes team has recommended pump therapy as a possible way to prevent further severe hypoglycemic events. Her parents have chatted with other parents on the internet and have expressed an interest.

Is Lauren a good candidate for pump therapy?

Later in this chapter, we will see how each of these youngsters did with pump therapy.

Getting Ready To Pump

The best way to prepare for a pump is to practice the skills required for success. Monitoring more frequently, calculating before taking carb/meal doses, and making high blood sugar adjustments are all skills needed when you go on a pump.

In our Diabetes Center in Houston, we put children and teens on intensive insulin management prior to beginning pump therapy. During this time, the child or teen uses multiple injections of Ultralente and Humalog. They begin to use insulin to carbohydrate ratios, test out flexibility in the meal plan, and use the 1800 Rule to calculate doses needed to lower high blood sugars. During this time, the child or teen learns how important it is to count carbohydrates correctly, dose insulin correctly, and record the information needed to make future decisions.

The transition from intensive insulin management to pump therapy is smoother than beginning pump therapy from a program based on 2 or 3 shots per day. After all, many of the concerns and questions about manipulating meals and snacks, doses, and testing are answered when learning intensive therapy. In addition, the diabetes team has a better idea of the starting basal and bolus doses which this child or teen will need.

This pre-pump program also allows parents to assess their child or teen's commitment to a more intensive approach to diabetes care. An added benefit to the family and team is that these children or teens can easily and safely be started on pump therapy in the outpatient setting. Insurance companies like that!

During this pre-pump time, it is a good idea for the parents and child or teen to understand the investment in time and money needed for pump therapy. The costs of pump therapy are discussed with them as well as the steps in the process.

Pump Training

Finally, you have your pump, you have all your supplies, and you have an appointment to learn how to use it all.

Any child or teen going on pump therapy must have at least one adult around who is trained in its use. The child or teen's primary caregiver must acquire the same skills the pump wearer does: setting basal rates, calculating and giving boluses, troubleshooting problems, preparing infusion sets, and assessing sites.

Other caregivers also must be considered. Whether the diabetes educator or physician trains these individuals or the parent or pump wearer trains them, they all must have appropriate knowledge of pump care. Babysitters, school nurses, camp nurses, and coaches need to know the basics: what a pump is, when and how to stop the pump (or at least how to remove the infusion set), the symptoms and treatment for hypoglycemia and hyperglycemia, and who to call for further help.

Setting The TDD, Basals, And Boluses For Children And Teens

Selecting an initial pump program for children or teens is not terribly different from the procedure for adults. However, there are a few differences to consider:

Children and teens often have a more pronounced Dawn Phenomenon than adults. Because of early morning surges of growth hormone, growing children and teens often need additional basal insulin in the predawn hours. Some may need an overnight basal rate that is higher than the daytime rate. Frequent nighttime blood sugar monitoring is necessary to determine whether the Dawn Phenomenon is present and its severity. Use these blood sugar results to determine whether and when increased basal rates are needed.

Children and teens often require one or two snacks, in addition to their three meals, to provide enough calories for growth. How to best cover these snacks needs to be considered when setting basal rates and boluses.

Teens have notoriously inconsistent daily routines and eating patterns. While the pump is the ideal tool for such a lifestyle, it initially will require that they keep a consistent schedule to set insulin doses correctly.

The hormones of puberty often challenge any insulin program. Hormonal changes can make this month's insulin program obsolete next month. Expect to change doses frequently. It is unlikely that the starting insulin doses will be perfect.

Setting The Total Daily Dose (TDD)

See Chapter 9 for a full discussion of setting TDD. A child's TDD always is determined before basals and boluses, which then are calculated as percentages of the TDD.

We know that certain guidelines suggest that the pumper begin pump therapy by decreasing the TDD used on injections by 25%. This may not be appropriate for teens. In fact, some teens need 100% or more of their pre-pump totals. Those who may need 100% include teens who have not had adequate blood sugar control before pump use, those who need to increase the food they are eating for growth, and those who have had wide blood sugar fluctuations.

Setting And Testing The Basal Rate

See Chapter 10 for a full discussion of setting and testing the basal rate.

Even though they often have a Dawn Phenomenon, we prefer starting children and teens with the simplest approach, a single basal rate. We then gather blood glucose data by testing the basal rate and making adjustments as needed.

Many guidelines recommend starting a pumper with 50% of their TDD as basal. This may be too low for teens. Our experience suggests that many teens need closer to 60% of their TDD as basal due to the level of circulating pubertal hormones.

One of the basal rate adjustments we make for a child or teen who often forgets to bolus for snacks is to increase the basal rate for two hours at snack time so that they don't have to remember to bolus. However, they must remember to snack.

Setting And Testing Carb Boluses

Chapter 11 has a full discussion of setting and testing boluses, and gives a good presentation of using the 500 Rule for Humalog to get the correct insulin-to-carb ratio.

We sometimes use another approach which is simpler but not as exact or flexible. We divide the number of carbs in the meal plan by the amount of TDD left over after the basal is figured. For example, if the TDD is 60 units and we use 60% for the basal, that leaves 24 units (60 units times 40%) for boluses. If the child has a meal plan with a total of 195 grams of carb in the day (breakfast=45, lunch=60, supper=60, and snacks=30), then 24 units must cover 195 grams of carb. We divide 195 by 24 and get 8.1, so 1 unit covers 8 grams of carbohydrate or about 2 units per 15 grams of carb, which we call a carb choice. For some people, this is simpler than counting carbs, but it's not as flexible when a set amount of food must be eaten at each meal and snack.

During testing of the insulin-to-carb ratio, we may allow a carb snack of 8 to 15 grams to be "free," which means the basal covers the snack without using a bolus. This will keep the pumper from getting too much insulin while we are still testing. Also the bedtime snack is not covered completely, especially during testing. For instance, for a 32-gram bedtime snack, we let the first 8 grams of carb be "free" and only cover the 24 remaining with an 8 (rounded from 8.1) ratio. So 24 divided by 8 = 3 units, one unit less than normally taken for a 32-gram snack. This protects against nighttime lows if the child or teen's exercise or activity level has been sporadic or inconsistent. Larger snacks need to be counted fully in the bolus amounts.

Be sure the child or teen work several sample problems using their insulin-to-carb ratio to see whether they understand how to determine their bolus for various foods and snacks.

Timing boluses: Usual guidelines suggest that when using Humalog insulin, boluses should be given 5 to 15 minutes before the meal. Boluses of Regular insulin are normally given 30 minutes before the meal. There are times, however, when the timing of the bolus must be individualized.

Pre-meal bolus: Basically, give the bolus before the meal when you are certain of the food you will be eating and the time.

Interim bolus: Sometimes it is safer to use a "bolus now, bolus later" approach. This is useful when you don't know how much food you will be eating or the time it will be available or served. This might happen during parties, restaurant dining, or all-you-can-eat buffets. It could happen also during holiday feasting, snacking on chips and salsa before the meal, or expecting to eat more that you really can (the "my eyes are bigger than my stomach" phenomenon).

After-meal bolus: This approach calls for a meal dose given immediately after the meal. It is especially useful for small children who may have unpredictable appetites or for anyone during sick days

Setting And Testing High Blood Sugar Boluses

See Chapter 12 for a complete discussion of setting and testing high blood sugar boluses. Have the child or teen determine how far he or she drops on a unit of insulin and test it to be sure.

Preparing For Pump Start Day

It is important to know what your diabetes specialist wants you to do with your insulin doses on the day before the pump start. If your pre-pump program includes Ultralente insulin, that insulin will need to be stopped 12-24 hours before the pump is started. If your pre-pump program uses a bedtime dose of NPH or Lente, it may be appropriate to have that dose the day before the pump start.

On the day of the pump start, you probably will not need an intermediate or long-acting insulin. When we start pumps, we encourage the child or teen to have breakfast after taking the morning quick-acting insulin (Humalog or Regular). Then it's off to pump class. By lunch, they are on the pump and bolusing for that meal. Use the *Instructions For Pump Start* form on page 46.

Roles And Responsibilities

The pump is a great tool, but it carries responsibilities. It is wise to discuss the roles of parent and child or teen with your health care team. In general, the diabetes care team should provide thorough training and complete recommendations for the insulin program. After the pump is started, that same team should be available for frequent consultation, especially in the first few days after starting the pump. While the pump manufacturers can assist with questions about the mechanics of pump use (such as alarms, infusion supplies, pump programming), they cannot offer clinical management such as dose adjustment. Your diabetes team is the best resource for questions in medical management.

Be sure to have close phone followup initially. In the first few weeks, basal rates will need to be adjusted. Even ratios of insulin to carbohydrate may need to be altered. Some centers use a system of faxed or emailed reports every few days. The most important information includes basal rates, boluses given and the time, amount of carbohydrate eaten and the time, and when a high blood glucose bolus was used. Some teams also will want to know the total daily dose infused for each day, exercise patterns, and dates of site changes.

If you are new to reviewing blood glucose log books, here is a simple system to highlight patterns of blood glucose levels. Use three different highlighter pens. First choose the target range for blood sugars. For example, if the target range is 80-150 mg/dl, for all blood glucose levels below 80 mg/dl, highlight the number with blue. For values between 80 and 150 mg/dl or in the target range, highlight with yellow. And for values over 150 mg/dl, use a pink highlighter. You will be able to see patterns quite readily.

For another method of recording, use the *Smart Charts* discussed in Chapter 6 They are a handy, convenient record that has everything that affects your blood sugar on one day on the same page. They also have a place for you to graph blood sugars, which is an excellent way to see any problems in your blood sugars, such as when you are too high or too low.

Initially, it is important to test the basal rates. That means the fasting blood glucose and the glucose levels between meals should be within target. If not, then the basal rate should be adjusted. See Chapter 10 for testing basal rates to see if they are correct. Once the basal rate or rates seems correct, work on the bolus ratio. The chart should help you to determine which part of the pump program is working at which time of day.

Evaluating Outcomes

How well pump therapy is working will depend on the individual reasons that the child or teen chose pump therapy. For example, if the goal was for fewer hospital admissions, then clearly the measure of success is number of hospitalizations. Other measures of pump success are based on different goals.

Are the child or teen and the parents happy with the program? How often do they report complaints or problems with the pump, the infusion sets, or the insertion sites? Has the child or teen explained the pump to friends and relatives? Has the child or teen benefitted medically?

Let's see how the three young people (Sally, Ralph, and Lauren) described at the beginning of this chapter have done on pump therapy.

Sally

In addition to her parents, Sally brought her best friend, Rachel, to her pump start. Sally, her friend, and her parents had carefully reviewed all the pre-training materials. Her pump training included a focus on use of the temporary basal rate. Because of her very active athletic and school schedule, Sally recognized that this feature would be immediately useful.

Within 2 weeks of starting the pump, Sally was able to make basal and bolus adjustments with guidance from her parents and her diabetes team.

At her next doctor's visit, Sally reported that she was extremely happy with her new therapy. What she liked best was taking fewer injections and not getting hypoglycemic during athletics. She also liked not having to eat before exercise. She did say that at times she was busy and forgot to bolus, but, she commented, "Rachel is there to remind me!"

Sally's HbA1c was 6.9 % at her visit.

Ralph

Because Ralph had had 2 recent DKA admissions, he needed a simple approach to pumping that allowed for his forgetfulness and provided frequent motivation and followup. His dietitian worked with Ralph to record and evaluate all the food he ate over a 3-day period. After analyzing his food intake, it became clear that Ralph generally ate the same amount of carbohydrate at about the same time each day. Based on that, Ralph's boluses were kept consistent with 10 units at breakfast and 15 units at lunch and supper.

Special care was taken when calculating Ralph's basal insulin needs. Ralph wanted to continue his afternoon and bedtime snacks. His basal rate was therefore set to cover these snacks without the need for a bolus dose. This insured that Ralph would have adequate insulin without having to remember to give a bolus.

Ralph's diabetes team worried that he might not be terribly conscientious about site care. To somewhat insure that sites would be changed frequently, the team insisted that he load his syringe with a set amount of insulin (only enough to last 3 days). This meant that Ralph had to do a complete syringe and infusion set change every 3 days.

Ralph's followup included phone contact every 3 to 4 days and visits every 2 weeks with his diabetes team. After the first 6 months of pump therapy, Ralph had no significant improvement in his HbA1c value. However, he had not been hospitalized and had not missed any school. Ralph prefers using the pump because he considers it more convenient. His diabetes physician agreed to sign Ralph's sports physical if Ralph continued to follow through with his part of the treatment plan. Ralph is now on the high school varsity basketball team (a goal he had for himself).

Ralph is interested in improving his athletic performance. He and his diabetes team are now working on tightening his blood sugar control to meet his new goals for exercise endurance and strength.

Lauren

Lauren's parents have had a large role and great responsibility in her current pump regimen. Both parents attended the pump training session. Both parents shared in checking the overnight blood sugars, despite their busy professional careers. Lauren and her mom gave a presentation to her school nurse, including a handout on how to bolus and how to stop the pump if needed. They made a simple chart explaining Lauren's insulin sensitivity factor for determining blood sugar boluses.

Lauren's parents prepare her lunch each day. Inside her lunch box, they send a note totaling her carbohydrates for the meal and the insulin dose she should take to cover the meal.

Initially, Lauren, the nurse, and her parents were mildly anxious about Lauren bolusing at school. Their anxiety diminished when Lauren would hold her pump next to the phone as Mom or Dad listened to the confirmation beeps!

While Lauren's parents are involved in her pump therapy, Lauren is also involved. She cleans her insertion site and monitors her blood sugars. For safety her pump employs several features. Lauren's basal rates are locked so that she can not alter them. She has not been taught to unlock this feature, although her parents know how to do this. In addition, Lauren knows that her pump is not a toy and that her friends are not to push any buttons. Finally, Lauren does all her bolusing under supervision.

Since beginning pump therapy one year ago, Lauren has had no further severe hypoglycemia.

Clearly there are a variety of reasons that people choose pump therapy. For Sally, flexibility was most important. For Ralph, the pump helped remind him to pay attention to his diabetes and offered new sports opportunities. For Lauren, her safety and her parents' sense of confidence were crucial. In some of these pump wearers, overall diabetes control was improved. In others, even though glucose control did not change initially, other factors in the wearer's health and development improved. In all cases, strong social support, from parents, friends, and the diabetes team helped to make the pump experience a success.

Special Child Or Teen Issues

There are several areas that you as a child or teenager may have concerns about. The following guidelines in these areas may help reduce your concerns.

Growth Spurts

Growth spurts and the onset of puberty can signal a time of blood sugar upheaval for the teen. The hormones responsible for growth also cause glucose to be released. The pubertal hormones cause a type of insulin resistance necessitating increasingly higher doses of insulin. The timing of this glucose release can be fairly unpredictable making the control of blood glucose during adolescence a frustrating time. However, pumps allow the teen to make rapid dose adjustments.

Most children require a total of about a half unit of insulin per pound of body weight each day. Teenagers, on the other hand, can require up to one unit for each pound of weight. This extra insulin is not an indication that the teen's diabetes is "worse." It is simply a physiological need caused by normal growth. Even so, as a teen's overall total daily dose increases, his or her insulin-to-carbohydrate ratio and high blood sugar ratio will also need to be adjusted.

Identification Tags

While wearing ID tags has always been a good idea for the child/adolescent with diabetes, it is even more important for the pump user. The problem is the ordinary ones may not appeal to the child. Some newer tags are colorful sports bands complete with the medical insignia, and some jewelry stores are making more attractive bracelets. In any event, it is not enough to carry an ID card in your wallet. You really need clear identification that emergency people can easily spot. Don't leave home without it!

School

Key school personnel should know about the pump: what it is, what it does, what to do in case of emergencies. Many schools have "zero tolerance" when it comes to medications and gadgets (like pagers). To avoid any problems, the child or teen and parent should prepare the school nurse, coach, and teachers. Your diabetes educator or physician can write a letter introducing the pump to your school.

Check with your school officials about where they would like you to test your blood glucose. Sometimes, because of health regulations or school policies, it is necessary to do all diabetes care in the nurse's office.

Have a school kit filled with all your necessities:

- extra batteries
- extra pump syringe or cartridge
- extra infusion set
- insulin (Humalog or Regular)
- standard insulin syringe or insulin pen
- blood testing supplies
- low blood sugar supplies
- ketone test strips

See also the *School Care Plan For An Insulin Pump* on page 266.

Physical Exercise

The exercise in school P.E. classes is not necessarily planned or consistent. One day the child or teen may be playing a vigorous game of soccer, and the next day watching a movie. Consequently, you must decide whether to use temporary basal rate changes or to supplement with an additional snack.

Immunization

We don't often think about the effect immunizations may have on blood glucose. In some children and teens, blood glucose can be elevated for a few days following immunizations. Typically, it means setting a temporary basal increase.

Dating

To tell or not to tell? It is a personal decision. Friends and dates are often inquisitive about the pump. It may serve as an "ice breaker" to start talking about your diabetes. On the other hand, you may feel more comfortable concealing the pump (and your diabetes) for awhile. The pump can be worn under clothing, on a belt or waist band, or in hidden pockets - you may have to be creative about where and how.

One other possibility is to come off the pump for a date or an evening out with a friend. This is risky and carries some responsibility. You will need to test frequently and possibly carry an insulin pen to take boluses throughout the evening. It is best to talk with your diabetes team about these issues.

Alcohol

Drinking alcohol can have several adverse effects for teens on pump therapy. Aside from the moral or legal issues about alcohol, there are several diabetes control concerns. Alcohol may prevent the liver from releasing sugar during hypoglycemia. This leaves you without the regulator that usually kicks in to bring you out of a low, which can be quite dangerous. Also the symptoms of hypoglycemia can look like intoxication, therefore treatment can be delayed. Alcohol can impair judgment, which can make it difficult to recognize hypoglycemia, can affect the accuracy of dosing decisions, or can lead to giving a bolus accidentally more than once.

To stay in control and make the best decisions, consider these tips:

- Know the laws in your state about drinking
- Remember, you still have the choice to say, "No thanks!"
- If you plan to drink, be sure to eat carbohydrates before drinking!
- Limit the number of drinks by drinking slowly or alternating alcoholic with nonalcoholic beverages
- Never drink and drive
- Wear your Diabetes Identification

- Let friends know you have diabetes and how hypoglycemia might make you look or act
- Test your blood sugar before going to sleep: you may need an extra snack

Eating Disorders

With all the focus on food, it is not surprising that some diabetic teens have eating disorders. Most often these teens are young women who have a distorted image of themselves and who want to lose inappropriate amounts of weight. They may discover a quick weight-loss technique by continuing to eat what they want while decreasing their insulin doses. Soon blood sugar (and calories) and ketones will spill into the urine, resulting in weight loss but also in a very risky medical condition.

Parents and diabetes professionals must stay aware of teens who are overly concerned about food. These teens also typically have poor glucose control because they do not program basal and bolus doses appropriately (something that can be checked in the pump's bolus, basal, and totals history.) For teens with these behaviors, psychological assessment and intervention are imperative.

If you are using any of these techniques or think that you have problems with food and weight, seek professional help. Untreated eating disorders are very dangerous and even life threatening.

Athletics

Pumps are the ideal tool for athletes. Depending on the sport, it may be possible to keep the pump on while competing. Adjustments in carbohydrates eaten, the basal rate, or boluses may be made so that blood sugar control can be maintained. Often a temporary decrease in the basal rate is needed for longer activities. If so, this rate change should be programmed to start at least one to two hours before the exercise begins and should continue throughout the exercise. In addition, the temporary basal reduction will often be necessary after the exercise to avoid post-exercise hypoglycemia.

If you happen to test your blood sugar immediately after exercise, you may see an elevated level due to the action of adrenaline during exercise and especially during competitive sports. Do not immediately give a high blood sugar bolus for this reading! Within an hour, the blood sugar will often come back down as levels of adrenaline drop. Drink lots of water and retest in 60 minutes. If the blood sugar doesn't come down by then, give a high blood sugar bolus to correct the high reading. A continuous blood sugar monitor is ideal for monitoring blood sugar changes during and after exercise.

If exercise will last three hours or less, some athletes will give a bolus to cover part of the basal insulin that will be missed over that time before disconnecting from the pump. If the athlete has planned prolonged exercise, it may be necessary to reconnect every couple of hours to bolus the missed basal rate.

You may need to eat extra carbs before, during, and after the exercise to prevent hypoglycemia. Sports drinks or glucose gels are handy choices. This often does not need to be covered by a bolus.

Commonly used adhesive tapes may not be enough to hold the infusion set in place during periods of heavy perspiration. There are a variety of alternatives available, including waterproof tapes, skin adhesives, and occlusive tapes. See Chapter 5 for brand names of these products.

See Chapters 18 and 19 on exercise and the pump for systematic guidelines about adjusting basals, boluses, and carbohydrates for various types of exercise depending upon duration, intensity, and training. Teens who are interested in exercise may want to join the International Diabetes Athletes Association (1-800-898-4311), which holds an annual convention with information sharing, workshops, and group activities.

Menses

Some young women may experience drastic differences in blood sugar levels a few days prior to the beginning of their menstrual periods, or during the first couple days of their period. However, many teens do not have regular, predictable cycles until several months after the onset of puberty. Some have highs that require increased basal and bolus delivery, some will tend to have lows following it, and some will notice little difference around their cycle. It is helpful to record both menstrual and blood sugar history for future dosing decisions.

Many teens do not have regular, predictable cycles for several months after the onset of puberty. After you have your first period, start recording your periods even though they may be irregular so that you can see how they may affect your blood sugar. If you have regular cycles, you can anticipate this effect and can always consider where you are in the menstrual cycle as a possible explanation for control problems.

Camping

Diabetes camp is a great way to meet other children and teens with diabetes. And often, many of these youngsters, their counselors, and medical staff members are pump wearers! The American Diabetes Association maintains a listing of camps throughout the U.S., as does Children With Diabetes at www.childrenwithdiabetes.com.

Sleep-Overs

Initially, some parents and children may feel apprehensive about nights or week-ends away from home when on the pump. Having a sleep-over plan can help relieve some of this anxiety. It is difficult to predict which direction the blood glucose will go during a sleep over. With the excitement and extra snacks, blood glucose levels may be higher than usual. On the other hand, because the wearer is awake during usual sleep time, the extra activity may actually cause lower blood sugar levels. The only way to know for certain is to test!

Sleeping In On The Weekends

When you first begin pump therapy, your diabetes team is likely to ask you to follow a specific schedule of waking, eating, and sleeping while they are customizing your basal rates. It is important to know that your overnight basal rate will maintain a safe blood sugar through the night and into the morning. To check this systematically, test your basal rates as shown in Chapter 10. Test several times throughout the night, watching for changes in blood glucose levels. Test the fasting blood sugar and skip breakfast. Then test several times before lunch. If your basal rate is correct, the series of blood sugar results you have collected should have values that are similar. Only when this is achieved is it safe to hit the snooze button and go back to sleep!

Fast Foods And Restaurants

Fast food guides and restaurant carbohydrate guides are extremely useful when children and teens are eating away from home. Most chain restaurants have nutrition information available in pamphlet form or upon request. In addition, books are available that give specific nutritional values for items on the menu at many family and chain restaurants. See Chapter 7 on carbohydrate counting, along with Appendix A.

For high fat meals, it may be necessary to use the "bolus now, bolus later" approach. For example, a pizza meal may require an initial bolus to match the carbohydrate intake and a later bolus to match the digestion of carbohydrate slowed by the fat. Some pumps offer a feature that delays the bolus or spreads the bolus over several minutes or hours.

Most condiments, such as ketchup, dipping sauces, and bar-b-que sauce have carbohydrates that should be considered when counting carb grams. For instance, ketchup may contain from 3 to 5 grams of carbohydrate per teaspoon or packet.

Before intensive insulin management or pump therapy, few people counted the grams of carbohydrate in non-starchy vegetables. We now recognize how important this source of carbohydrate can be. Here are some guidelines for estimating the carbohydrate amount of vegetables (such as carrots, lettuce, or other nonstarchy vegetables):

1 cup raw (uncooked) vegetables = 5 grams of carbohydrate
1 cup cooked vegetables = 5 grams carbohydrate

Use these guidelines to count carbs on vegetable plates and at salad bars!

Considerations for infants, toddlers and the pump

Over the past two years, our group has begun using insulin pump therapy in certain very specific groups of toddlers. Parents and health care providers may want to consider pump therapy as an option for toddlers who experience frequent episodes of severe hypoglycemia, or for those who experience rapid and wide fluctuations in their blood glucose levels. Traditional injection programs may be frustrating and difficult to manage when toddlers refuse to eat, are napping, or when ill. Pumps can make these situations easier to handle, as well as eliminating hypoglycemia from variable insulin action after injection. Insulin pump therapy, unlike current long-acting insulins, provides continuous 24-hour predictable insulin delivery. However, pump therapy should not be considered the mainstay of diabetes management for all toddlers.

Choosing a pump, insertion sites/sets, and how to wear it

The parent and diabetes team need to focus extra consideration when choosing the pump and accessories for the toddler. Problems have been experienced by some pump users when attempting to deliver very small basal rates (0.1-0.3u/hr). Small mealtime bolus amounts are also needed, sometimes as small as a tenth of a unit for every 10 grams of carbohydrate. Infants and toddlers rarely need 0.5 unit for an entire meal.

Pumps today have several "lockout" features to help prevent overdoses from small curious hands. Safety features like these can be used to prevent accidental boluses and unwanted alteration of basal rates.

For toddlers, the preferred insertion site is the buttocks. Using the old adage "out of sight, out of mind," this decreases chances that the small child will "play with or pick at" their insertion sites. Consideration should also be given to whether the child is potty trained or not, as skin care and hygiene are pertinent to preventing skin infections, and soiled diapers complicate this issue. In choosing insertion sets for comfort, short, direct-entry 6 mm needles or catheter-type sets are preferred to longer, angled sets. A disconnect feature may be desired for bathing or dressing.

The pump itself must be kept out of the reach of the toddler. We have had good luck with two different methods, both of which place the pump between the shoulder area on the child's back. One method uses a toddler harness (the type used for toddler leashes) with a specially created pouch to hold the pump between the shoulders. The other involves creating an undershirt with a pocket sewn medially in the upper back between the shoulders, with a velcro closure at the top to prevent the pump from falling out of the pocket during the usual twists and tumbles common to a toddler.

Parents can facilitate pre-pump "desensitization" by using the child's buttocks for injections prior to pump start. We ask the parents to have their child wear either the toddler harness or undershirt, with the pocket filled with an empty pump or an old pager, for a week prior to connecting to the live pump.

Keys to success

A cooperative effort between diligent, well-educated parents and their diabetes team is critical for success with a toddler wearing an insulin pump. Basal and bolus rates used in toddlers are very different than those needed by older children. Doses need to be carefully monitored by a team that is experienced in working with small children. Extensive pre-pump education and evaluation should include carbohydrate counting, how to evaluate basal and bolus insulin needs, sick day management, and troubleshooting skills.

During initial pump training we ask that the parents arrange childcare for the day, so that they can come to the office and learn without distraction. The Nurse/Certified Diabetes Educator/Pump Trainer works extensively with the parents on using the basic and more complex features of the pump. The parents fill the cartridge or syringe with saline, insert an infusion set into their skin and wear the pump themselves for the next three days.

They receive written instructions of exercises to perform, including boluses to administer, fictitious blood glucose values that they need to respond to, and times to use temporary basal rates. They are instructed to fill new cartridges or syringes, program the pump, prime new tubing and insert new infusion sets daily for three days. The ultimate goal of these exercises is for the parent to gain safe proficiency in performing these tasks prior to the toddler being placed on the pump.

On "Go Live Day," the parents and child come to the office. We review the bolus and basal history in the pump memory. We review the parents notes regarding their "pumping experience" and any questions or problems they may have had. The parents demonstrate filling the pump with insulin, programming and priming the tubing. They then insert the infusion set into the child, and the connection of the child to the pump is made.

Babysitters and Daycare

Babysitters and daycare providers can be easily trained how to deliver a bolus. We recommend postmeal bolusing in toddlers who may be finicky, picky or unpredictable eaters. Parents should create simple worksheets that give instructions to their childcare provider regarding how to give a bolus. Instructions should also be included on when to immediately contact the parent, for instance if the site comes out, if the blood glucose levels are abnormally high or low, if the child is vomiting, etc.

It is not appropriate that the parent expect the babysitter or daycare providers to be as efficient or as competent in managing the child with diabetes and an insulin pump as they themselves are.

Parents of toddlers treated with insulin pump therapy **must be accessible at all times**. Any delay in response time can cause significant harm to a child as a result of ketoacidosis or severe hypoglycemia.

Expectations

Parents of the toddler living with diabetes and their diabetes team should have realistic expectations for age appropriate goals of control. The desire for 'tight control' or for HbA1c's of less than 7% for the infant or toddler, who is unable to perceive and treat their own hypo or hyperglycemia, is **dangerous**. Instead, parents and healthcare providers should evaluate other parameters of success: Does the child have fewer episodes of hypoglycemia? Are the fluctuations in blood glucose levels more controlled? Has their quality of life improved? Are the parents less fearful and anxious? Is the child growing and developing normally? If the answers to these questions are "Yes," then the child and family are successful pump users.

Just because a toddler is treated with pump therapy during his or her early years does not ensure that pump therapy is the best treatment for the entire lifetime. Some school-aged children with diabetes may want to discontinue pump therapy because they feel different or no longer want to be connected to the device 24 hours a day. Parents and healthcare providers should always be sensitive to the child's wants and desires, recognizing that pump therapy is merely one method of delivering insulin that can always be resumed later as the child matures.

Troubleshooting

The types of pump therapy problems for children and teens are not terribly different from those that adults on pumps experience. The difference is in the individual pump user's problem-solving skills. Developmentally, youngsters may not be ready to analyze pump problems. Children and teens can be taught the basics of alarms and troubleshooting, but they still need good supervision from a knowledgeable adult.

Parents need to know how to verify the pump's program, how to look for basal and bolus history, and how to respond to a pump's alarms. Parents should review these screens regularly. See Chapter 25 on how to troubleshoot unexplained highs.

Kids tend to be rougher on pumps than adults. This may result in damage to the pump's casing. Although pumps are pretty sturdy, they can break if mishandled. We know a youngster who cracked the display window on his pump when he jumped down from the school bleachers! It is always a good idea to keep the pump in its protective case.

Summary

For years, insulin pumps and kids were not considered a good match, but this is no longer the attitude. Now pumps are truly an alternative for children and teenagers. The decision to start pump therapy should be based on the concerns and goals of the child or teen, parents, and diabetes team. The child or teen certainly must "buy into" the therapy, and the program must take into consideration the individual abilities and needs of the child or teen with diabetes. We have seen pump therapy be successful and safe in the well-trained and professionally supported child or teen and family.

The biggest things are the easiest to do because there's less competition.

Cornelius Van Horne

Pregnancy

Three to four percent of all pregnancies are complicated by diabetes. Usually the complication is gestational diabetes that begins during pregnancy, often near the end of the second trimester or during the third trimester. In the United States, 90,000 women have gestational diabetes every year. Another 10,000 pregnancies occur annually in women who have Type 1 diabetes prior to conceiving. All 100,000 of these women have a compelling reason for controlling their diabetes--to promote the health and wellbeing of their unborn baby and themselves.

Pumps have been shown to be great tools for improved blood sugar control during pregnancy. However, the entire health care team must be aware of how pumps operate and use established pump protocols specific to pregnancy. These are critical for handling situations such as unexpected highs or alternative insulin delivery methods should the pump be disconnected.

This chapter covers

- Why blood sugar control is more important during pregnancy
- Why blood sugar control is more difficult during pregnancy
- how to use pump therapy to stabilize control during pregnancy
- Pregnancy management
- Gestational diabetes
- Insulin adjustments during pregnancy
- Avoiding ketoacidosis with Type 1 diabetes
- Carb adjustments during pregnancy--the Rule of 18ths

Complications Found In Pregnancy

For good health, a person with diabetes needs to keep blood sugar levels close to normal all the time. This control becomes even more important during pregnancy because only strictly controlled glucose levels can create the environment needed to produce a healthy baby. High blood sugars before conception and during the first eight weeks of pregnancy often are associated with serious birth defects. Also, high levels in the second and third trimesters may result in fetal complications and problems at birth.

First trimester complications include

- Birth defects
- Spontaneous miscarriage

The risk for these complications increases when Type 1 or Type 2 diabetes is present but poorly controlled before conception.

Second and third trimester complications include

- Premature delivery
- Delayed growth and development
- Large birth weight (more than 9 pounds), often requiring a Cesarean section
- Severe low blood sugars in the infant after delivery
- Respiratory distress syndrome
- Enlarged heart
- Low calcium level and tetany (jitters)
- Jaundice
- High red blood cell count

These complications may occur due to poor control in Type 1 or Type 2 diabetes.

One possible complication of high blood sugars during pregnancy is that the baby at birth does not have fully developed lungs even though it is full term and normal weight. Underdeveloped lungs often cause the baby to have respiratory distress or difficulty in breathing after delivery.

High blood sugars during pregnancy can also cause severe low blood sugars in the newborn. In the womb, the fetus produces large amounts of insulin to compensate for the mother's high blood sugars, and after birth, the baby continues to produce excess insulin for several days, triggering severe low blood sugars.

How Does Control Affect Complications?

Since 1949, blood sugar control has been directly linked to the survival of the infant. In that year, Priscilla White, M.D., reported from the Joslin Clinic in Boston that 18 percent of the babies of mothers with diabetes were stillborn or died shortly after birth. She also noted that "good treatment of diabetes" clearly improved the outcome.[78] In 1965, Jorgen Pedersen, M.D., studying pregnant women in Copenhagen, reported that those women who had none of the Bad Signs in Table 21.2, had a 6.9 percent rate of fetal and neonatal deaths.[79, 80] In contrast, in 130 diabetic pregnancies where one of these signs was present, the death rate rose to 31 percent.[81]

During the late 1960's and early 1970's it became clear that the higher the average blood sugar level of the mother, the higher the risk that the child would be lost near birth.

By the 1980's, the mother's blood sugars and the child's metabolic environment could be normalized through blood sugar testing at home. This helped reduce complications after the mother became aware she was pregnant. At the same time, birth defects emerged as a major cause of infant deaths in babies born to women with Type 1 diabetes.[82, 83] In several studies that looked at this problem, birth defects were found to occur in 4% to 11% of infants born to women with Type 1 diabetes, compared to a rate of only 1.2% to 2.1% in the general population.[83, 84, 85] Researchers and physicians realized that blood sugars in these women needed to be normalized sometime before conception because the child's organs were forming rapidly within the first eight weeks after conception, often before a woman realized she was pregnant.

Several researchers also noticed that higher HbA_{1c} values during the first trimester were associated with more spontaneous abortions than were seen in nondiabetic women.[86, 87] Interestingly, one researcher found that women with diabetes who have excellent control throughout pregnancy actually have a lower rate of spontaneous abortions than nondiabetic women.[87] An HbA1c that is normal or no higher than one percent above the upper limit of the normal range minimizes the risk of both birth defects and spontaneous abortions.

Table 21.1 Blood Sugar Goals During Pregnancy

Time	Whole Blood	Plasma
Before meals and at bedtime:	60-90 mg/dl (3.3-5 mmol)	65-95 mg/dl
1 hour after starting to eat:	120 mg/dl (6.7 mmol)	130 mg/dl
2 a.m.–6 a.m.:	60-90 mg/dl (3.3-5 mmol)	65-95 mg/dl

Note: Keep your HbA1c at least 20% below the lab's upper limit for normal for non-pregnant women (i.e., in the normal range for pregnancy)

The conclusion drawn from these early studies was that maintaining normal blood sugars throughout pregnancy reduces the risk of complications. Furthermore, women with Type 1 or Type 2 diabetes who plan to conceive should keep their blood sugars at the levels recommended for pregnancy prior to conception so that a tightly controlled environment exists from the day of conception through delivery. The best way to maintain tight control is to follow the specific guidelines given below and, when recommended, to use an insulin pump for optimal control. Of course, if a woman with

> **Table 21.2 Things To Avoid In Pregnancy, Dr. Pederson's Bad Signs:**
>
> 1. Ketoacidosis
> 2. Preeclampsia (also called toxemia of pregnancy: a combination of high blood pressure, headaches, protein in the urine, and swelling of the legs, usually late in the pregnancy)
> 3. Kidney infection
> 4. Neglect of prenatal care

Type 1 diabetes and her health care provider opt to use an insulin pump, this should be started 3 to 9 months before conception to allow adequate time to achieve good control on the pump and ensure good control at the time of conception.

Control Problems in Pregnancy

Blood sugar control is more difficult during pregnancy for several reasons. First, a pregnant woman's blood sugar is normally lower than a woman who is not pregnant. To mimic this, target blood sugars for the pregnant woman with diabetes are also lower and closer to the hypoglycemic range. HbA1c levels should be maintained within the normal range for pregnancy (i.e., a range that is 20 percent lower than the lab's upper limit for normal—each lab's normal range will vary). Another difficulty arises when nausea and vomiting caused by morning sickness make eating and insulin coverage more difficult. Also problematic are hormone changes and gradual weight gain throughout the course of pregnancy that cause insulin need to rise constantly.

Preparing for Pregnancy

If you have Type 1 or Type 2 diabetes, you should have your blood sugar levels under control before you try to conceive. Until your blood sugars are controlled, use adequate birth control. Low dose birth control pills appear to be both safe and effective. Once your HbA1c is in the normal range, you can discontinue birth control.

If you have Type 2 diabetes, you should discontinue any oral medications you use to control blood sugars prior to conception. An alternate method of controlling your blood sugars should be worked out with your physician.

Achieving excellent control before conception is necessary because the fetus begins to develop specialized organs and tissues as soon as the egg is fertilized through the first three months of pregnancy. This development phase determines more than anything else whether the baby will be normal. High blood sugars interfere with cell division and can lead to DNA damage and birth defects. There is a 20 percent chance that the infant will develop complications or die if control is achieved only by the second trimester.[88]

If you are planning a pregnancy, you can benefit from eating healthy, exercising regularly, and supplementing your diet with a vitamin/mineral capsule designed for pregnancy. If you have diabetic complications such as damage to the eyes, kidneys, or vascular system prior to pregnancy, you have a greater risk of complications in pregnancy for yourself and the baby.[89] This does not rule out a healthy pregnancy but should be taken into consideration before pregnancy begins.

Pregnancy Management Program

Every effort should be made to keep your sugar normal throughout pregnancy. (See Table 21.1 for targets.) You need to manage your pregnancy in the following ways:

- Frequent blood sugar and HbA1c tests to determine the exact level of control
- Wear a continuous blood sugar monitor for around-the-clock monitoring
- An eye exam for retinopathy
- A 24-hour urine collection for creatinine clearance, total protein, and microalbumin to assess the health of the kidneys, done each trimester
- An evaluation of the cardiovascular system
- A detailed diet program, using the Rule of 18ths (see Table 21.4).
- A regular exercise program

Gestational Diabetes

The most common form of diabetes during pregnancy is gestational diabetes. It usually develops late in the second trimester or early in the third trimester of an otherwise normal pregnancy due to an increasing demand for insulin production. The current recommendation is that all pregnant women be screened with a shortened glucose tolerance test. This is routinely done in pregnant women between the 24th and 28th weeks (the sixth month) of pregnancy.

Women at high risk for gestational diabetes include those who are overweight, have a history of multiple stillbirths and miscarriages, have previously delivered babies weighing more than 9 pounds at birth, have had gestational diabetes previously, or have a strong family history of diabetes.

If you are high risk and are attempting to conceive, you should have a glucose tolerance test before conception. Then you should have another test as soon as pregnancy is confirmed, and testing should be repeated at 24 to 28 weeks of gestation if the first test was negative. These tests are done to detect a blood sugar problem as shown by a fasting serum glucose above 105 mg/dl (5.8 mmol) or a blood sugar above 140 mg/dl (7.8 mmol) at two hours after a meal.

Serum and plasma glucose values are 10% to 15% higher than whole blood values. Some home blood sugar meters measure whole blood, while others measure plasma values. See Table 21.1 for target blood sugar values for each.

Insulin Adjustments During Pregnancy

If you have well-controlled Type 1 diabetes, when you become pregnant, you will begin adjusting your normal basals and boluses as needed. If you have Type 2 diabetes, you may be controlling your diabetes with diet and medication. When you become pregnant, if you are on a diabetes pill, the medication is replaced immediately with insulin, since oral agents may have a negative effect on the fetus. If your diabetes is diet-controlled, your blood sugars should be monitored carefully at home and in the clinic according to the targets in Table 21.1. If you are likely to need insulin later during the pregnancy, your physician may want you to start on an insulin pump before it becomes absolutely necessary in order to familiarize you with its operation. If not started then, insulin will be started whenever the blood sugar rises above the targets required for a healthy delivery.

Insulin requirements rise steadily during pregnancy, usually doubling by the end.[84] This rise is caused by several factors—weight gain, increased caloric intake, creation of new tissue, and an increase in hormones made by the enlarging placenta that conflict with the actions of insulin. Each woman's experience varies which means an insulin program will be tailored to individual need. You should maintain a very strict regimen of blood glucose monitoring done at least eight times a day to alert yourself and your health care team quickly to your increased need for insulin. You should check before each meal, an hour after each meal, at bedtime, and at 3 a.m. The tests one hour after eating should be the highest blood sugar readings of the day. A test result in the lower end of the target range could indicate you should eat more carbs to avoid a low blood sugar. Table 21.3 shows the rise in insulin requirements throughout pregnancy for a woman with Type 1 diabetes.

Insulin pump therapy, with varied basal rates and boluses, works well for maintaining control in the face of a constant rise in need for insulin, especially in the last 4 months of pregnancy. You may need to raise your basal rates and boluses throughout the pregnancy. Allow 50 to 60% of the total daily dose for the basal rate and 40 to 50% for the carb boluses.

Because a high blood sugar overnight can damage the fetus if the pump fails, some healthcare providers have their patients reduce the overnight basal rate starting about two hours after bedtime and use an injection of long-acting insulin at bedtime to cover this reduced basal rate. This ensures that serious high blood sugars and ketoacidosis do not develop overnight if insulin delivery from the pump is interrupted for any reason.

Another option is to use a continuous monitoring device. It can be set to alarm whenever the blood sugar rises above 90 or 100 mg/dl (5-5.6 mmol) to allow the pump to be used alone for excellent overnight control.

For an immediate effect, you should use additional boluses when necessary to bring down a high blood sugar quickly so that the fetus is not harmed. If blood sugars continue to rise above your targets, it is time to raise your basals and boluses. Increased doses usually are required every 5 to 15 days through most of the pregnancy as determined by charting the blood sugars and the amounts of carbohydrate eaten. We recommend a graphical charting system, like *Smart Charts*, during pregnancy to track everything that may be affecting your control.

Table 21.3 Typical Increase in Total Daily Insulin Doses by Trimester*

If your weight is:	At this trimester: Pre	1st	2nd	3rd
100 lbs.	27 u	32 u	36 u	41 u
120	33 u	38 u	44 u	49 u
130	35 u	41 u	47 u	53 u
140	38 u	45 u	51 u	57 u
160	44 u	51 u	58 u	65 u
180	49 u	57 u	65 u	74 u
200	55 u	64 u	73 u	82 u

* Insulin requirements in many women with Type 2 diabetes or recently diagnosed gestational diabetes often start at these insulin doses, and may quickly increase due to the needs of the woman.

The need for insulin rises until the last four weeks of pregnancy when the fetus starts drawing out more glucose from the mother's blood for its needs. At this time the mother's insulin need may drop! To match this decreased need, reduce the basal rate and boluses. In particular, a reduced overnight basal and a larger bedtime snack often is required to keep the blood sugar from dropping during the night. Reduce your carb boluses as needed if you are unable to eat a substantial meal because of the enlarging uterus. However, if you experience a drop in your need for insulin not caused by these obvious reasons, contact your obstetrician for consideration of immediate delivery.

What if my sugar is high before a meal?

Take the carb bolus plus enough high blood sugar bolus to lower the high reading. Check the blood sugar every 30 minutes until it is below 120 mg/dl (6.7 mmol) before eating. If the blood sugar is still high two hours later, recheck your pump and take an additional high blood sugar bolus by injection. If you cannot delay eating, eat the fat and protein portions first and have the carbohydrate as late into the meal as possible to allow the reading to drop.

Ten to fifteen percent of women with gestational diabetes require insulin to control high blood sugars. You need insulin as soon as blood sugars rise above the range in Table 21.1. Insulin doses for gestational diabetes must be handled on an individual basis. Some women are sensitive to insulin, but many more are resistant. A starting point is to use total insulin doses similar to those found in Table 21.3. An insulin pump often is used in pregnancies involving Type 1 diabetes, but it may be equally helpful for insulin delivery during gestational diabetes.

How To Use Insulin When Nausea Occurs

Nausea and vomiting often occur in the first trimester. A pregnant woman with Type 1 diabetes may think that because she cannot eat when she's nauseous, she doesn't need any insulin. This is not the case. The liver continues making glucose and releasing it into the blood stream. Insulin is needed to keep the blood sugar from rising even if no food is eaten. The pump can be helpful during this part of the pregnancy, because the basal rate on the pump can be used to deliver insulin even if nausea prevents eating.

Glucagon should be kept available for use anytime the carb bolus has been taken for a meal that you find yourself unable to eat due to nausea. An injection of glucagon raises the blood sugar by causing the liver to release some of its stored glucose. Of course, if nausea is frequent, you may want to take only part of your carb bolus and then attempt to eat. If food can be eaten, you can take the rest of the bolus. If food or caloric drinks cannot be kept down, you may inject a partial dose of glucagon at that time to quickly raise the blood sugar.

Glucagon: How Much Do You Need?

Each 0.15 mg of glucagon (or 1/6 of the standard 1 mg. dose) raises the blood sugar 30 mg/dl! Avoid taking too much glucagon, as this raises the blood sugar too high and may cause nausea, which is what you are trying to avoid.

Ketoacidosis And Pregnancy

In Type 1 diabetes, the greatest threat to the fetus and the mother are high blood sugars leading to diabetic ketoacidosis. If the mother develops severe ketoacidosis, there is a 95 percent probability that the fetus will die. An insulin pump often is used to provide the strict control needed, but special precautions are necessary to insure that the pump and infusion sets are working correctly. The following precautions help to avoid ketoacidosis:

- Test the blood sugar frequently to ensure that insulin delivery is constant, or use a continuous blood sugar monitor

- Change the infusion set every 48 hours or more frequently, and always when an unexplained high blood sugar occurs. Avoid changing the set just before bedtime

- Give insulin by syringe or insulin pen, instead of by pump, to lower any blood sugar over 160 mg/dl (8.9 mmol)

- Check the urine for ketones every morning and when the blood sugar is above the target level

- Reduce the nighttime basal and use an injection of long-acting insulin to cover about half of the overnight pump basal

Carbohydrate Adjustments During Pregnancy

Eating a balanced diet is important for a pregnant woman with diabetes. Because the fetus is continually removing glucose from the mother's blood for growth, eating many meals and snacks throughout the day is also important.

During pregnancy, a diet comprised of 40 percent carbohydrate, 40 percent fat, and 20 percent protein is generally recommended. Spread the carbohydrate portion throughout the day to make blood sugar control easier. An easy way to spread these carbohydrates is by using the "Rule of 18ths." With the help of your dietician, estimate your total daily caloric need. Then distribute the carbohydrate portion throughout the day (see Table 21.4) based on the number of 18ths of total carb needed at that time.

As an example, if you require 1800 calories per day, eat 180 grams of carbohydrate. This total of 180 grams divided by 18 (Rule of 18ths) equals 10 grams per 18th. According to the table, your breakfast would include 20 grams of carbohydrate.

The breakfast carbohydrate is kept low in comparison to the rest of the day. Most women with Type 1 diabetes have at least a mild Dawn Phenomenon and therefore are more resistant to insulin at the beginning of the day. Women with gestational diabetes often have insulin resistance which can also cause high morning readings. Keeping carb intake low until noon helps in dealing with this. Since strict control is of such importance, staying away from high glycemic foods which can spike the blood sugar is a good idea at any time.

Your caloric need will rise during the pregnancy, usually adding a total of between 500 to 1,000 extra calories per day over the nine months. These calories supply fuel for your higher metabolic rate and your required weight gain. The distribution of carbohydrates changes along with the calorie change. Table 21.5 provides guidance for distributing the carb portion of these calories.

Table 21.4 Carb Distribution With The Rule of 18ths

Meal or Snack	Portion of The Day's Total Carbohydrate:	Percent of Total Daily Carbs
Breakfast	2/18	10%
Midmorning Snack	1/18	5%
Lunch	5/18	30%
Midafternoon Snack	2/18	10%
Dinner	5/18	30%
After-Dinner Snack	2/18	10%
Bedtime Snack	1/18	5%

Labor And Delivery

During active labor at the hospital, muscle contractions can be similar to strenuous exercise, thereby reducing insulin need dramatically. The goal is to maintain blood glucose levels between 60 and 100 mg/dl. To attain this, you may need to reduce your basal rate quickly and temporarily discontinue boluses. The pump may be taken off completely and an intravenous line started with insulin added as needed to lower the blood sugar and glucose added to raise it. Test your blood sugars hourly or have someone else test them to ensure that the pump or intravenous line is controlling the blood sugar.

After Delivery

After the baby has been delivered, the hormones in the placenta that antagonize insulin are no longer at work. Insulin requirements rapidly drop. Most women with gestational diabetes who require insulin during their pregnancy do not require it after delivery. The woman with gestational diabetes may continue to have diabetes and need treatment, but often she returns to impaired glucose tolerance or to normal blood sugars. Between 20% and 50% of women with gestational diabetes develop Type 2 diabetes, either immediately or sometime within the next 20 years.

The reduced demand for insulin after delivery, together with the prolonged "exercise" of labor, may be so dramatic that even in Type 1 diabetes insulin may not be needed for a day or two. If the woman has had a caesarean, her eating is limited for the next two to three days, which limits her insulin need also. In a few days, the woman with Type 1 will be back to her pre-pregnancy insulin requirements.

Table 21.5 Grams Of Carbs Through The Day Based On Daily Calorie Need

Meal	Carbs as 18ths	Total Calories Per Day							
		1600	1800	2000	2200	2400	2600	2800	3000
Breakfast =	2/18 =	19 g	20 g	22 g	24 g	26 g	29 g	30 g	34 g
Morning Snack =	1/18 =	9 g	10 g	12 g	14 g	14 g	14 g	16 g	17 g
Lunch =	5/18 =	44 g	50 g	55 g	60 g	66 g	72 g	78 g	82 g
Afternoon Snack=	2/18 =	18 g	20 g	22 g	24 g	27 g	30 g	31 g	34 g
Dinner =	5/18 =	44 g	50 g	55 g	60 g	66 g	72 g	78 g	82 g
Evening Snack =	2/18 =	18 g	20 g	22 g	24 g	27 g	29 g	31 g	34 g
Bedtime Snack =	1/18 =	9 g	10 g	12 g	14 g	14 g	14 g	16 g	17 g
Total Carbs/Day = 40% of total cal/day =		160 g 640 cal	180 g 720 cal	200 g 800 cal	220 g 880 cal	240 g 960 cal	260 g 1040 cal	280 g 1120 cal	300 g 1200 cal

Breast Feeding And Type 1

If you breastfeed (which benefits the baby's immune system), insulin requirements may be lower than before conception because more glucose is needed for breast milk. Adjust your calorie intake to match the child's breastfeeding habits. If the baby consumes most of its calories at bedtime or in the middle of the night, you must do the same. Many Type 1 women need only a low basal rate to cover eating in the evening with this breastfeeding pattern.

When I was a kid my parents moved a lot
— but I always found them.

Rodney Dangerfield

Pump And Site Problems

When unexpected high blood sugars occur, pump users too often assume it's because "I ate too much." Rather than scrutinizing the situation for all possible causes, they follow any food they've eaten along an easy path to guilt. The wise pumper keeps in mind that highs are often caused by mechanical failure of the pump or infusion set.

A problem with blood sugar control might be due to variations in carb intake, variations in weight, stress, a change in activity, an infection, or a change of schedule, but it may also be caused by any interruption of insulin delivery. It's important to quickly differentiate whether a high blood sugar is due to a mismatch between your insulin dose and lifestyle, or to an unrecognized problem with your site, infusion set, reservoir, or pump.

Mechanical problems cannot be solved by giving more bolus insulin. Assuming they can may easily lead to an unnecessary hospital bill. It's critical to recognize when the pump, infusion set, reservoir, or insulin is the source of high blood sugars.

In this chapter, we

- Identify technical and mechanical problems that occur during pump use
- Troubleshoot unexpected high blood sugars caused by a pump
- Show how to lower risks for pump problems
- Review when to call your physician/health care team

An insulin pump enhances your ability to maintain good control, but it is also a mechanical device that can itself cause problems. Proper maintenance and monitoring are needed to ensure that a pump will continue working. Typical pump problems will be encountered within the first six months of use, then will decrease in frequency as your experience grows. After you know how to troubleshoot unexpected high blood sugars, problems tend to become less frequent and less severe because you are in better control of your equipment.

Keep in mind that the first sign of a pump problem is usually an unexpected high blood sugar, rather than an alarm from your pump. When you encounter a high blood sugar, keep mechanical problems, site problems, and bad insulin in mind as potential sources for unexpected highs. See the information box on page 40 for information on spotting bad insulin, such as tiny particles or a yellowish color.

Pumps will sound an alarm if they have a clog or stop delivering insulin. That warning can help prevent a high if you troubleshoot the problem when you hear the alarm and check the alarm code for its source.

A good principle to use when solving a pump problem is start at the site and work back to the pump: Start with looking for an insertion set that has been pulled out, a lump under the skin (hematoma, scarring, or abscess), blood in the line, air in the line, loose or disconnected infusion set, damaged infusion line, loose hub, O-ring leak. Rule out each possible cause before going on to the next one.

Troubleshooting The Pump

An insulin pump is a mechanical device that can fail due to improper technique or defective parts. Pumps have audible alarms but only for some problems, which are outlined in the tables in this chapter. Keep your ears alert for pump alarms, but keep your eyes open for other causes of unexplained high blood sugars. A high blood sugar is seen within 2 to 4 hours if insulin delivery is interrupted for any reason.

If your blood sugars are unexpectedly high or are over 250 mg/dl (13.9 mmol) on two consecutive tests, take an injection to reduce the high blood sugar before trouble-shooting the pump. Remember: an interruption of infused Humalog insulin can trigger ketoacidosis within 4 to 5 hours.

Test your urine for ketones at the first sign of trouble. Do not assume nausea and vomiting are due to food poisoning, the flu, or another cause. If ketones are present in the urine at moderate or large levels or elevated in the blood, contact your physician/ health care team immediately. Ketoacidosis makes you resistant to insulin, and your doctor may recommend giving 50 to 100 percent more insulin than usual by injection for high blood sugars.

Check blood sugars hourly and drink a large amount of noncaloric fluids until corrected. A continuous interstitial glucose sensor allows easy tracking of how effectively you are lowering the high blood sugar.

Whenever you are unsure of the reason for high blood sugars, check to see what your total daily insulin delivery is, your last bolus taken, and your basal rate so that you are sure you have given all the insulin you assumed you had. Then take Humalog or Regular insulin by injection, replace the reservoir and infusion set, and use a new injection site as precautions.

How To Avoid Pump Problems

Common problems related to the pump and infusion set are listed in this chapter, while site and skin problems are covered in the next chapter.

Clogging

The most common causes for clogging are a low infusion rate, leaving the pump in suspend mode for lengthy periods, and bad insulin. If you have a low basal rate because you are sensitive to insulin, a diluent can be added to the insulin so the flow rate is increased. Discuss this with your physician if you feel it may help.

There are several other possible causes for clogged lines. Reuse of reservoirs and infusion sets increases the risk of clogging. Foreign materials, such as betadine or alcohol, may cause clogging if introduced into the reservoir or line. Hand lotions, hair sprays, or solvents on your hands, skin, clothing, or in the air may penetrate the infusion tubing and cause clogging. Always use special care when handling your insulin, syringes and infusion sets. If your tubing comes in contact with very hot water, as in a steaming shower or hot tub, the heat may coagulate the insulin. Always protect your insulin and infusion line from heat. Insulin is a protein just like an egg white…don't cook it.

If you try to give a large bolus through a clogged line, an alarm should sound on the pump. However, if you give only a small bolus or have only basal insulin passing through the line, the pump does not perceive a clog and an alarm will not sound until pressure has built up. Depending on the situation, this delay in warning could be several hours. Before you get an alarm to warn you, your blood sugar may already be high.

Most common sign of clogging is a high blood sugar or alarm.

Table 22.1 Clogs		
Information	**Causes**	**Solutions**
Insulin and the plastics in reservoirs and infusion sets are not totally compatible. When clogs occur, insulin comes out of solution and crystallizes, usually near the end of the infusion line, or out-of-sight inside the teflon tubing at the end.	May be a sign that insulin is bad. More likely when infusion sets are used beyond 3 or 4 days and with low basal rates.	Check that a clog is the problem by completely removing the entire infusion set with teflon tubing. After removal, give a 2 to 5 unit prime or bolus. If insulin comes out easily, a clog is not the cause, so check carefully for other sources for the high. If delivery is slow or nonexistent, a clog is likely. Replace the reservoir, infusion set and insertion set.
Will Pump Alarm? Yes		

Leaking

Insulin leaking from your reservoir or infusion set is difficult to see or feel. The amount of insulin lost is so small it is quite hard to detect, and your pump will not warn you of leaks. Insulin has a distinctive smell, like that of creosote, or railroad ties, or Band Aids, but regular blood sugar tests are the only reliable way to detect leaks. As with clogs:

Most common sign of a leak is a high blood sugar.

Table 22.2 Leaks		
Information	**Causes**	**Solutions**
O-rings		
A good seal between the O-rings and the reservoir wall is needed to keep insulin from leaking out the back.	When reservoirs sit in a warehouse or pharmacy, the lubricant needed for a tight seal between the O-rings will pool at the bottom of the reservoir.	Relubricate the O-rings before filling the reservoir with insulin. Use care in handling, especially while inserting the reservoir into a pump. Replace the reservoir, infusion set and insertion set.
Hub		
A snug fit is required between the infusion line and the reservoir to prevent insulin loss.	More common if the hand grip is weak, or when inattention occurs due to haste.	Look for fluid around the hub. Check for the smell of insulin. Try retightening gently with small pliers. If loose, this may be the problem.
Line		
Unusual, but can occur with any kind of trauma.	Catching in door or drawer, or from curious child or pet. Rarely caused by manufacturing defect.	Feel and look for any damage along the infusion line. After giving a bolus, check for any drops of insulin along the line. Replace the infusion set, reservoir, and insertion set.
Will Pump Alarm? No		

How To Check For Leaks And Clogs

If an unexpected high blood sugar occurs, remove the whole infusion set, including the insertion set and metal needle or Teflon tubing:

- Send a 10-unit bolus through the tubing to check for clogs. If no insulin appears at the tip, the infusion set is clogged. If insulin appears immediately at the tip, the infusion set is not clogged. If clogged, the 10-unit bolus should trigger a high pressure alarm or reveal a leak in the line. Check the infusion line, hub or O-rings for leaks. Insulin has an odor described as that of railroad ties or a bandaid. If insulin can be seen or smelled at the hub or is visible along the infusion line or between the O-rings, a leak is responsible for the high blood sugars.

• If neither a clog nor leak is present, consider other causes for high blood sugars.

Important Warning

Take an injection at any time that you experience a second consecutive unexpected high blood sugar. If you suspect any problem in insulin delivery, immediately inject Humalog or Regular insulin by syringe. After the injection, replace the complete infusion set and reservoir, using fresh insulin. Place a new insertion set at a new location. Check the blood sugar frequently until you are sure the problem has been corrected. Drink plenty of fluids, more than you feel you need.

Ketoacidosis and subsequent hospitalization are twice as common among people using pumps compared to those using injections. Never assume it won't happen to you. Most cases could be avoided by following these simple steps.

Tunnelling Of Insulin

The skin, like any other organ, rejects foreign objects like Teflon and metals. After an insertion set is placed through the skin, the surrounding tissues will at first have a mild inflammatory reaction with a little bit of swelling. Normally, this isn't even noticed by the person wearing the pump. As time passes, however, and the Teflon or needle stays in place, surrounding tissues begin a healing process that hardens the surface along the foreign material. The increased speed of this process next to an inert substance like Teflon, or perhaps the greater flexibility of the Teflon itself, allows a small path to form along the length of the Teflon or needle. Then, with any movement of the set itself, especially an active game of golf or tennis, the gap becomes large enough that insulin begins to leak from the tip of the insertion set back to the surface of the skin. Once this begins, control becomes impossible with this insertion set.

To our awareness, no research has been done regarding this problem, but a number of pumpers who are active have complained about it, particularly when using shorter, 90-degree Teflon insertion sets. On occasion, a drop of insulin will be clearly visible following a large bolus around a set's entry point if it has a window to visualize this area. It will also occasionally happen with metal needles, but appears to be less frequent because of their lack of flexibility or a longer inflammatory response.

Most common sign of tunnelling is a high blood sugar.

Table 22.3 Tunnelling		
Information	**Causes**	**Solutions**
Blood sugars rise unexpectedly due to leakage of insulin along Teflon infusion set or metal needle back to the surface of the skin. More common with Teflon insertion sets, especially those inserted at 90 degrees, or after prolonged use. Very common after 6 or 7 days. Often seen following activities like golf or tennis.	Because Teflon is inert, it may encourage tissues beside it to "heal" and harden. Bumping or movement of the infusion set then loosens contact between the teflon and tissue, and opens a path for insulin to escape to the outside surface.	Use insertion sets no longer than 3 to 4 days. If this happens frequently, try using angled Teflon or 90-degree metal needle infusion set. Replace the reservoir, infusion set and insertion set.
Will Pump Alarm? No		

Running Out Of Insulin

Today's reservoirs hold 300 units of insulin, but many pumpers forget how quickly this insulin disappears. The following tips help in managing your insulin supply:

- Keep an insulin bottle and syringe or an insulin pen available at all times.

Plan ahead so you don't run out of insulin at an inconvenient time. Keep a regular schedule for changing your infusion site and filling your reservoir. Choose a convenient time and change your site every third or fourth day at that same time. Change your infusion set in the morning to avoid having a dislodged needle or other mechanical problem go undetected for several hours during sleep.

- If you have used more insulin than usual, and don't have enough in your reservoir to last until your next scheduled change, conserve your pump insulin by using it only for your basal. Temporarily use injections from a syringe for your boluses. Just make sure there is enough insulin left in your reservoir to provide the basal insulin you need.

- If you run out of insulin in your reservoir and have no other insulin available, remember that a pump with an empty reservoir has 17 to 25 units left in the infusion line.

- Your pump has a built-in alarm to warn you when your reservoir is nearly empty, usually with 20 units remaining. When you hear the alarm, start planning how to deal with it.

Table 22.4 Other Pump Problems

Problem	What To Do	Pump Alarm?
Infusion Line Not Primed	Problem appears shortly after changing infusion set. Look for large lengths of air in line. Replace infusion set entirely or disconnect from insertion set and prime line. Can cause DKA or major control problem. Be very careful with preparation technique.	No
Empty Reservoir	Check to see if your reservoir is empty and replace. Arrange set changes on a regular schedule to prevent this from occurring unexpectedly.	Yes
Dislodged Insertion Set	Look at insertion site carefully. If loose, replace insertion set and/or infusion set and reservoir.	No
Incorrect Programming	Usually occurs after reprogramming the basal rates. Check your basals for correct starting time and correct rate. Reprogram as needed.	No
Dead Battery	Replace battery. Some batteries, such as silver oxide ones, last longer.	Yes
Mechanical Problem	These are rare. Pumps will detect electronic problems and give an alarm. Other problems, like worn threading on the plunger driver, will provide no warning, but can be detected with testing.	Yes/No

Summary

Whenever your blood sugar is high, sort out in your mind whether there is a clear cause for it, such as extra carbohydrate intake, too little bolus or basal insulin, an infection, etc. If there is not a clear reason for the high reading, use Tables 22.1 through 22.4 to check for mechanical causes.

Always remember that frequent blood sugar testing will warn you of serious problems before they become serious.

Do not continue to rely on pump therapy if your blood sugar remains high and you are unable to correct it. Anytime your blood sugar readings are over 250 mg/dl (13.9 mmol) twice in a row without a good reason, take a conventional injection of Humalog or Regular insulin and test your blood sugar more often to make sure you have corrected the problem. Replace your syringe and entire infusion set before continuing use of your pump. Check your urine for ketones; call your physician/health care team immediately any time you find your ketones are moderate or high, as this can quickly deteriorate into severe ketoacidosis.

Little minds are interested in the extraordinary; great minds in the commonplace.

Elbert Hubbar

Skin Problems

An infusion needle is like a splinter or any other foreign body placed under the skin. It can cause irritation, discomfort, or infection. Allergic reactions can be caused by adhesives used on infusion sets, surfactants on infusion needles, the metals in metal needles, or more rarely by insulin itself. Some pumpers have no difficulty with skin problems, while others have to pay close attention to avoid them or treat them.

Who is likely to develop skin problems? No one really knows. No clear relationship exists between how well blood sugars are controlled and skin problems associated with pump use. The wisest approach is to follow safe techniques to reduce your risk.

This chapter discusses how to deal with these infusion site problems:

- Tape allergies
- Infections
- Bleeding
- Pump bumps
- Pump hypertrophy

Allergies

Your skin may not accept every tape or dressing you use to keep the infusion set in place. A particular tape may cause an allergic reaction. This problem is relatively easy to diagnose because you will notice that the itchy area, irritation, or redness on your skin patterns itself after the shape of the tape or dressing.

If you are allergic to tape or adhesive material, the allergy usually starts a few days or weeks after the tape is first used. To cope with an allergy, simply switch to another brand of tape, adhesive dressing, or infusion set. One tape that generally sticks well is Micropore™ skin tape by 3M. If a problem occurs with white Micropore™ tape, there is a brown, hypoallergenic Micropore™ tape that is less likely to cause allergies. Silk tape or Hypafix tape also can be tried.

Another treatment for a tape allergy is to use a protective dressing, such as Skin Prep™, on the skin before applying the tape. This product provides a protective barrier between the skin and the offending tape and can often reduce or prevent the risk of an allergic reaction. Discuss using Skin Prep™ or changing to another tape with your physician/health care team.

Adhesive materials can also be interchanged. IV 3000, Johnson and Johnson Bioocclusive Material, Tegaderm and others can all be tried. Allergies can also be triggered by the plastic infusion line which is easily identified by the red snakelike pattern it leaves behind where it contacted the skin surface. Skin Prep™ or a non-offensive adhesive material can be placed under the infusion line as a barrier. If teflon or a metal infusion set are the culprit, there are fortunately a wide variety of infusion sets made by different manufacturers that can be tried.

Insulin allergies are usually associated with itching and redness at the infusion site. An insulin allergy can trigger widespread and serious problems like anaphylactic shock, but fortunately insulin allergies are extremely rare with today's highly purified insulins.

Infections

The risk for infection is greater when using an insulin pump than when using injections. Most infections result from poor technique, such as breathing onto the infusion set, not washing your hands with soap and water before starting to change the set, touching the infusion needle or top of the insulin bottle, not using IV Prep™, Betadine™ Solution or Hibiclens™ on the skin, not using a bio-occlusive material, or leaving the infusion set at one site longer than 72 hours. A good way to prevent infections is to be conscientious about using the sterile technique described in Chapter 5. Assuming infections will happen will make you take extra care that they don't.

Watch for these signs of an infection at the infusion site:

- redness or inflammation
- warmth
- pain
- swelling

If any of these signs occur at the infusion site, contact your physician/health care team immediately. Recognizing an infection early usually allows easy treatment with an antibiotic. If treatment is delayed, an infection can develop into an abscess and require surgery or hospitalization.

Your physician will be far happier calling in a prescription for you than having to lance an abscess or write hospital admission orders. You also will be assuring your physician that you are a well-informed, well-trained pump user when you call at the first sign of this potentially serious problem. Do not wait until it has become a crisis.

When an infection starts, it can spread to a new infusion site. If you have an infection or suspect one, remove the infusion set you are using and start taking your insulin by injections with a syringe, using proper sterile technique. Use a new infusion set at a new site only after you have started an antibiotic.

Bleeding

Bleeding from a broken blood vessel can occur whenever an infusion set is placed through the skin, but actually, bleeding is infrequent. It may create a cosmetic problem or, at worst, require changing the set. Bleeding can occur in three areas, and each requires different treatment.

On Top of the Skin

This is noticed as blood stains beneath the tape or dressing. When an infusion set is inserted, it can nick a small blood vessel near the surface of the skin. This surface bleeding can be ignored as long as the site is not inflamed, painful, enlarged, or threatening to discolor your wardrobe. Monitor this situation carefully to make sure it doesn't worsen. Even though this situation isn't critical, moving the infusion site ensures that further bleeding will not occur.

Inside the Infusion Tube

This is noticed as blood inside the infusion tubing near the needle, and means that bleeding is occurring at the tip of the infusion set. This type of bleeding under the skin may dilute the insulin the pump is delivering, decreasing its action. A high blood sugar may be the first sign of this problem. Whenever you see any blood inside the infusion tubing, immediately remove the infusion set and place a new one at another location.

Under the Skin

Bleeding under the skin may cause a lump under the skin called a hematoma. If you touch the infusion site, you can feel a hard lump about the size of a quarter underneath the needle. It may feel uncomfortable or sore in the same way that a bruise does. The skin may be normal in color or slightly red. Bleeding into the infusion tubing or around the needle on your skin may accompany a hematoma.

A pool of blood under the skin dilutes the insulin the pump is delivering, and a high blood sugar may be the first sign of this problem. When you check for problems, you will find a hard, enlarged spot under the skin. A pool of blood like this is an invitation for bacteria to grow and multiply, thus increasing the risk for infection around the infusion catheter or needle, which is a foreign body. If bacteria are present, they can multiply within the hematoma and cause an abscess.

Move the infusion site immediately if you have a lump under the skin at the infusion site. Firmly squeeze the lump to extract as much as you can. If the discharge comes out bright red, it is most likely a simple hematoma, but if any other color is seen, it is likely an abscess requiring an antibiotic. Monitor the site carefully. If you have any doubts or questions about whether a sore spot is a hematoma or an infection, call your physician/health care team immediately. Early treatment is always best.

Pump Bumps

A pump bump sounds like a dent found in your pump after you've dropped it. Instead, it is a slightly red, raised, pimple-sized spot found at the infusion site after the infusion set is removed. It often itches. After changing the infusion set and moving the needle to a new site, the bump gradually disappears. There are several theories about the causes of pump bumps. These include a reaction to the coating on the outside of the needle or catheter, or a reaction to preservatives and other trace chemicals found in insulin.

If you are concerned about pump bumps for cosmetic reasons, there are a couple of ways to reduce the chance of getting one. Cover the infusion site with IV Prep® and place an IV 3000 or other adhesive on the skin before inserting the infusion set. Take extra care to use sterile technique, and change the infusion site every 48 to 72 hours. Teflon catheters reduce the likelihood of pump bumps.

Hypertrophy At The Infusion Site

Some pumpers find that after using their pump for some time, a slight enlargement occurs in the area of the body where the infusion needle is placed. Hypertrophy is a medical term that describes this enlargement (atrophy is its opposite), so this problem is called pump hypertrophy.

Pump hypertrophy is caused by the higher concentrations of insulin placed under the skin at the infusion site. Extra insulin causes cells, especially any fat cells, in contact with the insulin to grow. This is not a medical problem, although some find it a cosmetic concern. Don't be alarmed if you notice hypertrophy in the area of your infusion sites. Discuss this with your physician/health care team if you feel it is a problem. If pump hypertrophy or pump bumps occur at an infusion site, avoid this area for 3 or 4 weeks. Temporarily switch to other areas of the body, such as the buttocks, to allow healing to occur. Be sure to rotate your sites over a wide area to lessen the risk of pump hypertrophy, and be sure to change to a new site twice a week, regardless of whether you see a problem or not.

Poor Absorption At Infusion Site

Poor site absorption from scarring seems to receive more of the blame for control problems than any other single cause, but if all the other sources for high blood sugars are carefully looked at, scarring at the site rarely turns out to be the real cause. A quick way to eliminate tissue scarring as the cause of high blood sugars is to ask, "How soon after I put my new insertion set into place did the high blood sugar occur?" If the blood sugar begins to rise within two or three hours of inserting the new set, poor absorption becomes one of several possible causes, but if the blood sugar problem starts 8 or more hours later, definitely look for another explanation for the high reading.

If certain parts of your anatomy seem firm and unyielding to touch, or have undergone surgery or experienced an abscess in the past, these will not be the best locations to place your infusion sets. Luckily, skin is our largest organ and offers many opportunities.

Never go to bed mad. Stay up and fight.
Phyllis Diller

Patterns
And What To Do

Blood sugar patterns are simply any consistent repetition of your blood sugar readings. For instance, a so-called "normal" pattern would be waking up almost every morning with your readings between 70 and 120 mg/dl (3.9 to 6.7 mmol), while an abnormal but consistent pattern would be waking up almost every morning with a reading over 200 mg/dl (11.1 mmol). On the other hand, the absence of a pattern would be waking up with your blood sugar being anywhere between 30 and 300 mg/dl (1.7 to 16.7 mmol) on any particular morning.

By recording your blood sugar levels daily and reviewing a few days or a week's worth of charts at a time, you can usually see certain patterns start to appear. Plotting the pattern of readings from a continuous interstitial glucose monitor on a graph or via a computer program, and then comparing the shape of these curves from several days' readings will help you see your patterns and give you insight into the effectiveness of corrections you try. Often, doctors can spot the patterns you may miss simply because they have seen so many charts before. Identifying problem patterns in your readings is the first step toward correcting them.

This chapter will show you

- Typical problem patterns
- Various ways to correct them

Patterns may be consistent and occur almost every day or for several days in a row, or they may be random and occur only occasionally but be connected to a certain event. When trying to spot and correct patterns, it is important to have a consistent schedule of times you eat and sleep each day. An erratic lifestyle usually leads to erratic readings. A bit of consistency often can let you determine what action you need to take, and it can help you deal with your blood sugars during erratic schedules as well.

Be sure you really understand how your insulin, basals and boluses actually work, because this information lets you adjust your insulin properly to your lifestyle.

Test frequently and record what you eat, especially grams of carbohydrate, basals and boluses, and activity.

Below are samples throughout one day. Blood sugars become a pattern if you see the same general levels repeat several times over a few days in a row as you review your charts. It is an occasional pattern if it occurs only as a result of specific choices you make, such as eating bean burritos for dinner.

Some people's daily activities or food patterns are so varied that it is hard for them to see any patterns. For better control, they will need to take the time to be consistent in one aspect long enough to see just what the blood sugar does under that circumstance. Once that problem is improved, isolate another aspect for study.

Suggestions for improving them are given below each pattern. For repeating patterns (i.e., high all the time or often low in the afternoon), insulin dose adjustments are usually needed. For occasional patterns, use a one time fix that can be reused in the future when needed. The blood sugar ranges on the left of the charts are given in both mg/dl (U.S.) and mmol (Canada, Europe, etc.) values.

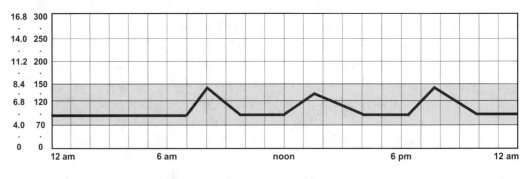

Pattern: Normal

Action: Nothing, keep up the great work!

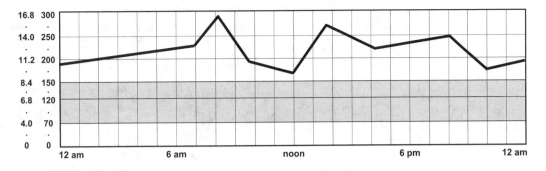

Pattern: High

ACTION: Raise your TDD, both basal rates and boluses. Review your diet, exercise, and weight, and make any improvements. Consider whether infection, pain, stress, bad insulin, steroid, or new medication may be causing the high readings.

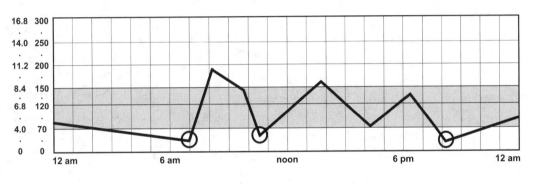

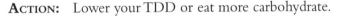

Pattern: Low

ACTION: Lower your TDD or eat more carbohydrate.

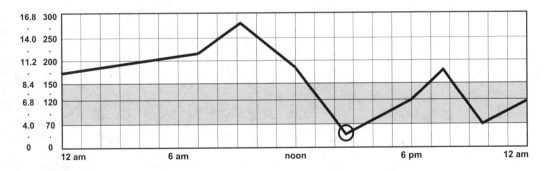

PATTERN: HIGH TO LOW—using high blood sugar boluses to lower highs that are too large for later control

ACTION: Recalculate your point drop per unit using your TDD and 1800 Rule (Table 12.1). Review the unused bolus rule (Table 13.1); test more often and be sure to eat if your blood sugar starts dropping.

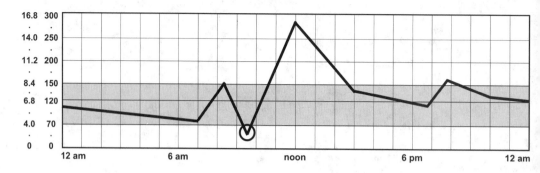

PATTERN: LOW TO HIGH—eating too much for low blood sugars

ACTION: Use only glucose tablets or fast carbs for lows, and eat less. When more carbs are eaten than are needed, take at least a partial bolus to cover the excess carbs. **Remember:** one gram of glucose raises your blood sugar 3 to 5 points.

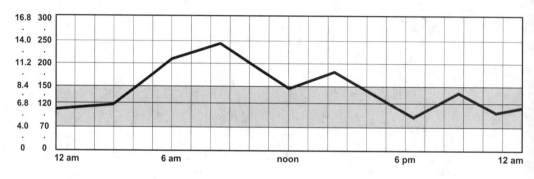

Pattern: Dawn Phenomenon

ACTION: Increase your basal rate gradually, starting about five hours before waking and lower it two or three hours after waking.

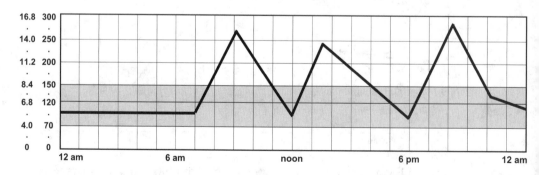

Pattern: Highs Between Meals

ACTION: Raise your basal rate slightly two or three hours before the meal; take your bolus earlier. Split meals or snacks into smaller portions; eat foods with a lower glycemic index or add high-fiber items (psyllium, guar gum) to meals.

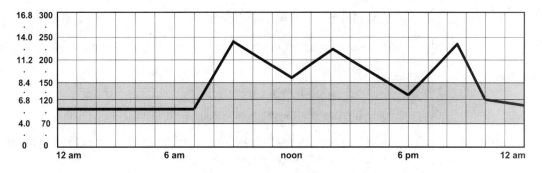

Pattern: Highs After Meals

ACTION: Raise your carb boluses (fewer carbs per unit of insulin); eat less carbohydrate; exercise after the meal; take Humalog carb bolus at least 20 or 30 minutes before eating, being careful to watch for premeal lows.

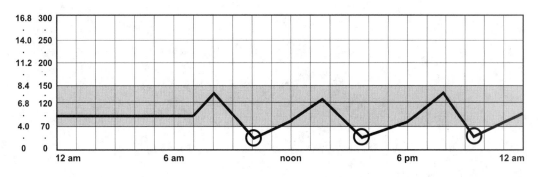

Pattern: Low After Meals

ACTION: Reduce your carb bolus (more carbs per unit of insulin); increase carbohydrates.

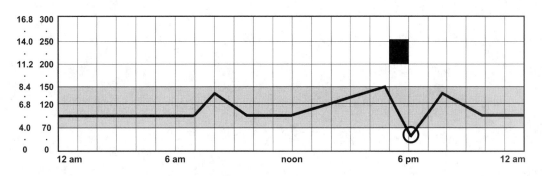

Pattern: Exercise Lows

ACTION: Reduce your basal rate two hours ahead of longer exercise, reduce meal boluses and/or increase carbohydrates right before exercise.

A Checklist For Pattern Control:

1. What is your target blood sugar before and after meals, and at bedtime?

2. Are you testing 4 or more times a day, or using a continuous glucose monitor?

3. Are you recording your blood sugars, carbs, boluses, and exercise?

4. Are you looking for the patterns in your test results?

5. When a problem pattern appears, can you identify how your basals or boluses need to be adjusted, or can you recognize a lifestyle change that might correct it?

6. Have you tried adjusting your bolus or basal insulin doses?

7. Did this adjustment improve or worsen the problem?

Searching for simple answers rarely uncovers the truth.
Instead, it leads to superstition, prejudice, panic, and war.

K.C. Cole

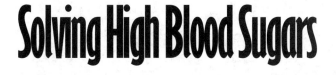

CHAPTER 25

Solving High Blood Sugars

The first blood sugar of the day is the most important one for determining the entire day's control. It's often the hardest reading to bring into the normal range, especially if you have a Dawn Phenomenon or Type 2 diabetes. Waking up with a high blood sugar after going to bed with a normal reading can be very discouraging.

In this chapter, we'll explore

- Causes for highs before breakfast
- Causes for highs at other times
- How to correct them

Highs Before Breakfast

Why does a high morning blood sugar throw off the rest of the day? Most often, when the breakfast reading is high, it is caused by a low insulin level in the blood. In the nondiabetic, a low insulin level occurs when the blood sugar is also low. When the liver senses a low insulin level, it responds by releasing sugar into the blood. In diabetes, the liver responds the same way to the low blood insulin level, but here the blood sugar is already high! Once the liver starts producing glucose, it is difficult to stop. Extra sugar continues to be produced and released through the morning hours.

Whenever you need an extra bolus for a high morning blood sugar, be careful of afternoon lows, especially when two or more high blood sugar boluses are taken during the morning and at lunch. In this situation, an insulin reaction later in the day becomes likely. Gorging on food in the panic of an insulin reaction can cause the blood sugar to rise again, with the cycle repeated. High morning blood sugars that result in this cycle often throw off control for the rest of the day.

Five common causes for high blood sugars before breakfast with corrections are presented.

Too Little Overnight Basal

Blood sugar may rise during the night because the overnight basal rate is too low. Too little background insulin is present to keep the blood sugar controlled.

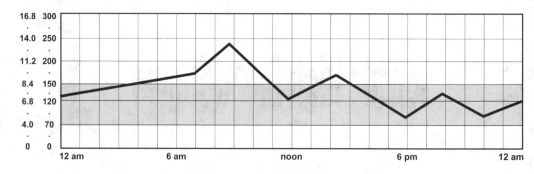

Test: Bedtime: Normal blood sugar.

2 a.m.: Usually midway between the bedtime and waking sugars.

Waking: Always higher than the 2 a.m. and bedtime readings.

If you frequently get these test results, your high morning blood sugar is caused by too little nighttime basal.

Action: Raise the evening basal rate about 9:00 p.m. and return to normal about 7:00 a.m. to provide more overnight coverage. You may wish to review Chapter 10 and test a new dose. Be cautious when raising your nighttime basal! If you've had nighttime reactions in the past, discuss this carefully with your physician. As you adjust, test blood sugars more often, especially at 2 a.m.

A High Protein Dinner

This pattern is similar to the Too Little Overnight Basal Pattern above, but it only occurs occasionally rather than consistently, and its cause and treatment are different. When protein is eaten, 40 to 50 percent of it will change slowly into glucose over a period of several hours following the meal. The amount of protein in most meals has little influence on blood sugar levels. When large amounts of protein are eaten, however, the blood sugar often rises overnight. Examples of heavy protein intake would be an 8 to 12-ounce steak, a Mexican dinner with a lot of refried beans, or an evening snack of several ounces of nuts.

Test: Bedtime: Normal blood sugar

2 a.m.: Usually midway between the bedtime and waking blood sugars.

Waking: Always higher than the 2 a.m. and bedtime readings.

If you typically get these results after a high protein meal or snack, the protein is causing your high morning blood sugars.

Action: 1. Limit the protein in evening meals.

2. Consider raising the basal rate slightly over a 6 to 8-hour period on evenings that you eat high protein meals to offset the increased glucose produced from the protein. Cover any high bedtime readings with a high blood sugar bolus, using half of your usual bolus if you want to avoid a nighttime reaction.

3. If necessary, wake up halfway through the night, check your blood sugar, and correct it with a smaller than normal bolus if it is high.

From your past experience you often can predict that a particular high protein meal will raise the blood sugar overnight. You then adjust your evening basal rate only on the nights you eat this high protein meal. If you can't predict the meal's effect, you may want to wake in the middle of the night and correct the blood sugar then, if necessary. If your experience is limited, testing at 2 a.m. is the best way to avoid a nighttime insulin reaction, or a high morning blood sugar.

High Bedtime And Morning Blood Sugar

This pattern is easy to identify because the blood sugar is high in the morning only because it was already high the night before at bedtime.

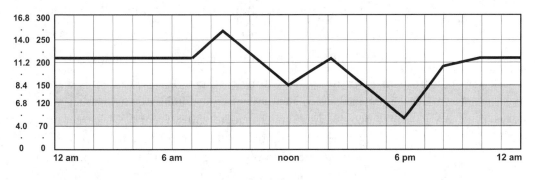

Test: Bedtime: High

2 a.m.: High

Waking: High

Test results show that the blood sugar was already high when this person went to bed.

Action: First, be sure the overnight basal rate has been tested and correctly set. Fully cover any carbohydrate eaten during the evening hours with a bolus. If the blood sugar is high at bedtime, take enough bolus insulin to bring it down but not enough to cause a nighttime reaction. Be sure to use the unused bolus rule in Chapter 13 to estimate how much bolus is still working from the dinner injection. Test the blood sugar at 1 a.m. or 2 a.m. to prevent a nighttime low blood sugar. If you are keeping your bedtime reading high because you are concerned about having a reaction during the night, discuss this situation with your physician/health care team.

The Dawn Phenomenon And High Morning Readings

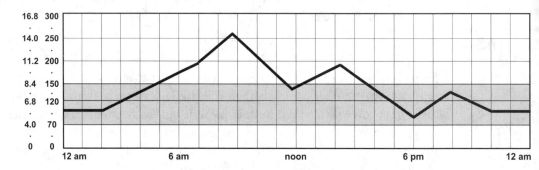

The Dawn Phenomenon pattern shows the need for a higher basal rate in the early morning hours. Ideally, the basal rate would rise between the hours of 1 a.m. and 3 a.m. to prevent this early morning rise (for those who sleep typical nighttime hours).

Test: Bedtime: Normal blood sugar.

2 a.m.: Close to bedtime blood sugar, much lower than the waking reading.

Waking: Much higher than the 2 a.m. and bedtime readings.

Test results point to a high morning blood sugar caused by a Dawn Phenomenon.

Action: Increase the nighttime basal rate. The best effect is seen when you raise the basal one to two hours before the blood sugar usually starts its own rise. For people with Type 1 diabetes, 50 percent to 70 percent need some extra insulin beginning between 1 a.m. and 3 a.m. to control the Dawn Phenom-enon. About 20 to 30 percent need substantially more insulin to keep the breakfast reading controlled. Be sure to check with your physician/health care team to make sure you have a Dawn Phenomenon before increasing your nighttime basal rate.

Although a true Dawn Phenomenon does not occur in Type 2 diabetes, a high morning reading is often a problem. Type 2s are not susceptible to insulin reactions at night so they can use a higher basal at bedtime and then increase it at 1 or 2 a.m. to cover the tendency to go high in the morning.

The reason for the high morning readings in Type 2s is somewhat different than Type 1s. People with impaired sensitivity to insulin, as often is true with Type 2s, tend to release more fat into the blood during the night when eating has stopped. Fat makes cells less sensitive to insulin, and because the liver begins to think that insulin levels have dropped, it starts to make glucose to raise the blood sugar even though it is already high! Due to these crossed signals, the liver creates unneeded glucose and causes the person to wake up with a high blood sugar.

To prove this, someone with Type 2, who finds themselves in this situation, can try eating a long-acting carbohydrate, like a green apple or raw cornstarch, at bedtime. This keeps the liver from producing glucose and will often help lower a slightly elevated morning reading.

Overtreating A Nighttime Insulin Reaction

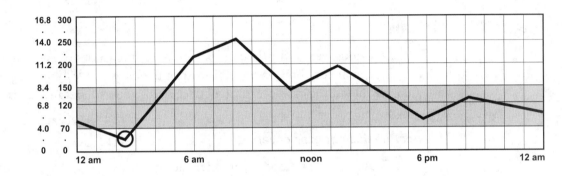

It's hard to be rational when you wake in the middle of the night feeling the effects of stress hormones released during an insulin reaction, especially when brain cells aren't getting enough fuel to think clearly. Because of the fear and confusion that follow, emptying the refrigerator may seem normal and reassuring. Overeating in the wee hours, however, results in sky-high blood sugars the following morning, and these often last for several hours into the day.

Test: Bedtime: Varies; can be low, normal or high.

2 a.m.: Low to very low, followed by excessive eating (over 25 to 30 grams of carbs)

Waking: Always high after eating too much for the low.

These results suggest that this high morning blood sugar is caused by overtreating a nighttime insulin reaction.

Action: The best solution is to determine why the nighttime reactions are occurring and prevent them. Lower the evening basal rate, the dinner bolus, or any high blood sugar bolus given in the evening if one of these doses is the culprit. The second-best solution is to keep glucose tablets or other quick-acting carbohydrate beside the bed and use it routinely to treat all nighttime reactions. Even in the middle of the night, it is hard to overdose on glucose tablets. A small amount of cheese or other protein can provide additional insurance against another low.

Frequently (half the time in most research studies) people do not wake up during a nighttime reaction. If someone sleeps through a nighttime reaction, the morning blood sugar will rarely rise any higher than 150 mg/dl, unless the basal rate for the early morning hours is too low.

If you have high blood sugars in the morning and are blaming them on reactions during the night, test your blood sugar a few times at 2 a.m. to find out what is happening. Also see Chapter 15 for the signs that unrecognized nighttime lows may be occurring. For more information on setting and testing basal rates that work to control blood sugars during the night and all day, see Chapter 10. If you are having problems with high morning blood sugars, you may want to reset and test your basal rates.

Highs After Meals

In the previous part of this chapter, we looked at the causes of and remedies for high blood sugars before breakfast. In this part of the chapter, we'll look at people who have a normal blood sugar before a meal but then lose control because it rises sharply after eating.

This part of this chapter covers

- Causes for high blood sugars after eating
- How to correct these highs
- Unrecognized nighttime reactions as a cause for post-breakfast highs

The last example is specific to breakfast, but the other remedies can be applied to any meal of the day that results in a high afterward.

Carb Bolus Missed Or Too Small

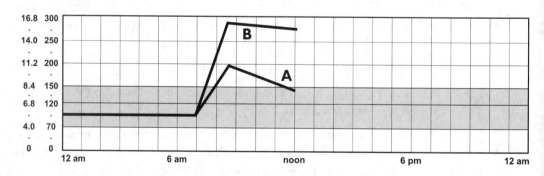

Here the carb bolus taken before a meal was too small for the carbohydrate eaten (line A), or was missed entirely (line B).

What happens: You can frequently underestimate the ratio of insulin to carbohydrate if you don't count your carbs. Even if you count carbs, at times you might misjudge the bolus to take for a meal, such as in a restaurant. In most cases when this pattern occurs, too little insulin has been taken for the food. Forgetting to take a bolus is—hopefully—a rare occurrence.

Action: Retest your ratio of grams of carbohydrate to each unit of Humalog to be sure that you are getting the right bolus for your meals. Also review Chapter 7 on carb counting to be sure you have a good understanding of this excellent tool. At many restaurants, nutritional information is available to guide your doses. A little attention to meals that consistently give you problems will lead to a solution.

If forgetting a bolus occurs often, try changing your pattern of bolusing, perhaps taking it while the food is being prepared rather than in the bustle of sitting down to eat. If you do that, be sure your blood sugar can hold you that long or eat fruit or other carbs right after bolusing.

Carb Bolus Taken Just Before Eating

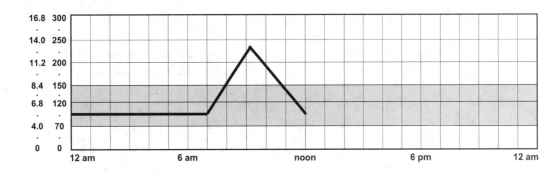

What happens: This problem is more common with the use of Regular insulin but is occasionally seen with Humalog. Regular insulin takes at least 20 to 30 minutes to have any effect and at least 2 1/2 to 3 hours before it peaks in its activity. In contrast, carbohydrate creates an almost immediate rise in the blood sugar. When a bolus of Regular is taken just before a meal, the carbohydrate raises the blood sugar before the Regular has a chance to counteract it and a high blood sugar follows. This high blood sugar will return to normal before the next meal because the insulin finally has its desired effect.

This pattern is common when boluses of Regular are taken just before meals. How high the blood sugar goes depends on the person's sensitivity to insulin, the amount of carbohydrate eaten, any activity after the meal, and the glycemic index of the foods eaten.

Action: Be sure to use a fast insulin like Humalog in your pump, and try to bolus 20 minutes before the meal. With Regular, take the bolus 30 to 45 minutes before eating. If unable to take your bolus early, try one or more of the following:

- subtract carbohydrate from the meal and use it later as a snack,
- add fiber like psyllium or guar gum to the meal to slow down the digestion of carbohydrates, or
- get extra exercise just after eating.
- use the medication acarbose (Precose) before the meal to slow down the digestion of carbohydrate.

A Fast-Acting Carbohydrate In The Meal

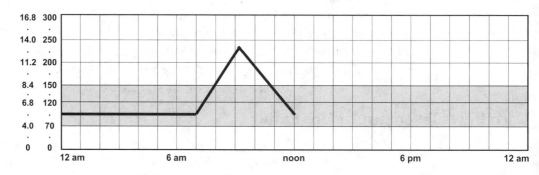

What happens: This pattern is similar to the last one. But instead of a bolus that's taken too late, here a fast-acting carbohydrate causes the blood sugar to spike before the carb bolus taken for the meal can enter the blood. Many foods have a high glycemic index. That is, they raise the blood sugar quickly after meals, even though no more carbohydrate than usual is eaten.

If you eat 70 grams of carbohydrate for breakfast as old-fashioned oatmeal, your blood sugar isn't likely to rise dramatically. If you eat a typical cold cereal, it probably will. Many typical breakfast foods, like cold cereal with a ripe banana, instant oatmeal, yogurt with a fruit syrup, or a toasted cheese sandwich, will spike the mid-morning reading. This is much more likely with Regular than Humalog, but it can happen with Humalog.

Use of a continuous glucose monitor will enable you to quickly see the action time of different foods, and how high the blood sugar peaks with each.

Action: Check the glycemic index of the suspected food in Appendix B. Partially or totally replace the fast-acting carb with slower ones—those that have a low glycemic index—such as old-fashioned oatmeal, high-fiber cereals, strawberries, or plain yogurt with fresh fruit sliced into it.

Other possible solutions:

- With Humalog, take the carb bolus 20 to 30 minutes before meals that contain fast carbs, being careful to watch for premeal lows and not delaying the meal.

238

- Eat less carbohydrate for the meal; then add a carbohydrate snack a couple of hours later

- Add fiber like psyllium or guar gum before the meal

- Get extra exercise after the meal.

- Use the medication acarbose (Precose) before the meal to slow down the digestion of carbohydrate.

All of these problems, too little carb bolus, a bolus taken too close to the meal, and fast carb foods can occur at any meal of the day. The solutions also can be applied to any meal of the day. The next situation is more specific to the breakfast meal.

An Unrecognized Nighttime Reaction

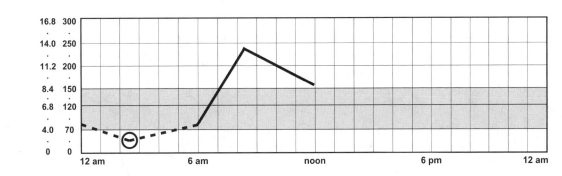

What happens: This pattern is typical for the morning hours following an unrecognized nighttime reaction and is due to a significant release of stress hormones during the reaction. Notice in this pattern that the blood sugar often may be normal before breakfast. Review Chapter 15 for signs of nighttime reactions.

   This pattern occurs even when someone correctly covers the breakfast carbohydrate with a carb bolus. The action of the usually adequate bolus is blunted by the stress hormones released during the nighttime reaction, and the blood sugar rises. Stress hormones can raise blood sugar levels for 8 to 10 hours after a major reaction. The blood sugar may remain high at lunch and into the afternoon.

Action: Learn to recognize the symptoms of a nighttime reaction. Try to determine the cause of the reaction and correct the evening insulins if necessary. Check your blood sugar at 2 a.m. if you're not sure of the cause. As an ounce of prevention, it's smart to do a 2 a.m. or 3 a.m. test every two weeks even when you're not having any problems.

   Setting the alarm feature on a continuous blood sugar meter will warn you every time your blood sugar drops below the limit you set, while a download of the data into a PC lets you see the entire night's readings.

Do not squander time, that's the stuff life's made of.

Benjamin Franklin

Variable Blood Sugars

Variable blood sugars can happen even on an insulin pump. Though a pump provides the best opportunity for stable, normal blood sugars, it does not guarantee this. When looking at blood sugars, variable is hard to define. Most people would be annoyed by blood sugars that frequently stray outside the 70 to 140 mg/dl range before meals and beyond 200 mg/dl after meals, particularly when they see no reason for the unexpected numbers. If your blood sugars show very little pattern when they go up and down, they could be considered variable. Before deciding that, though, you need to look closely for causes you might be missing. If you can spot them, you'll be able to have better control.

Let's be clear. If blood sugars are often high at one time of day, such as at bedtime, this is not a variable pattern but a rather consistent, abnormal pattern. When blood sugars are consistently abnormal, the cause is usually easy to identify. It may be that the carbohydrate bolus is too small for the evening meal, there's a problem with snacking after dinner, or the evening basal rate is set too low.

Blood sugars that are truly variable, on the other hand, have little identifiable pattern to them, but careful analysis often will uncover causes that can be identified.

Some factors that cause variable blood sugars include

- Insulin reactions
- A variable lifestyle
- Problems with certain carbohydrates or foods
- Stress
- Problems with the infusion site

Questions To Ask If Your Control is Poor With No Apparent Pattern:

If you see no apparent pattern in your blood sugars and your control is not what you would like, check all the following characteristics that apply to your management:

• Frequent or severe low blood sugars?	yes	no
• Erratic eating (different carbs, different times)?	yes	no
• Skipped meals?	yes	no
• Insulin doses that change a lot from day to day?	yes	no
• Exercise that varies in timing, duration, & intensity?	yes	no
• No exercise at all?	yes	no
• Irregular sleep hours?	yes	no
• Stress?	yes	no

If you answer "yes" several times, your control could be improved by dealing with these areas of your life. For instance, if your life is rather random, try introducing more regularity into it to prevent lows and lessen stress. Your charts then will begin to have a recognizable pattern to them. If this pattern does not conform to the control you would like, at least you then can analyze it for solutions.

Insulin Reactions

Frequent insulin reactions can trigger variable blood sugars. If too much insulin is being taken or if the reaction is overtreated in a panic, variable blood sugars result. If a high blood sugar occurs because the reaction was overtreated and extra bolus insulin is needed, this increases the risk for another reaction. The key to good control is to stop the lows first.

Pattern:

Insulin reactions as a cause of variable blood sugars are easy to recognize on charts: frequent low blood sugars that are followed 1 to 4 hours later by highs. When low blood sugars are followed by blood sugars above 150 mg/dl, overtreatment is likely. If these highs are often followed in the next few hours by another low, too much insulin is being given, usually in the high blood sugar bolus used to bring the blood sugar down.

What To Do:

• Start by reducing your TDD by 10%, as described in Chapter 14. If uncertain about how to change your insulin, contact your physician/health care team immediately.

• Use glucose tablets or quick-acting carbs for all reactions. Glucose tablets relieve symptoms faster than anything else and can be measured precisely which helps prevent overtreatment. Glucose or dextrose tablets can be obtained from many pharmacies and from most of the mail-order diabetes supply stores.

• If you don't have glucose tablets, use another fast-acting carbohydrate or simply reduce the amount of carbohydrate you use. For most reactions, 15 to 30 grams of any fast-acting carbohydrate will bring the low blood sugar quickly back to normal. Fifteen grams is the equivalent of a cup of milk and one square graham cracker, two-thirds of a small banana, or 4 to 5 ounces of a regular soda. Take only 15 grams and then in 20 minutes, after brain function has improved, retest your blood sugar. At that time, determine whether or not you really need more carbohydrate.

If you are wearing a continuous glucose monitor, watch for the effect of the 15 grams on your blood sugar. Take more if the original 15 grams does not appear to be raising your blood sugar.

• If you can't stop yourself from overeating, calculate the total amount of carbohydrate you have eaten and subtract the amount needed to cover your reaction. Then cover the excess carbohydrate so that you won't get a high.

Variable Lifestyle

People are usually aware of how consistent their lifestyle is. Whether or not you eat and sleep at regular times and get exercise on a regular schedule is easy to recognize. Whether or not work or school schedules are consistent is also important to recognize.

In determining basal rates and boluses, it helps to have a consistent lifestyle. If you have an irregular lifestyle and variable blood sugars are occurring, create as stable a lifestyle as you can to sort out the causes. Then, if necessary, go back to your previous schedule, using caution and taking the time to analyze what might be having a negative impact on your control. You can counter this impact once you know its source.

Pattern:

The lack of a pattern is the pattern.

What To Do:

• Carefully test and chart your blood sugars seven times a day, together recording stress, exercise periods, general health, etc. (See *Smart Charts* in Chapter 6)

• Eat meals with the same amount of carbohydrate and at the same time of day for awhile.

• Exercise regularly and consistently. Note whether the type, amount or timing of exercise has variable effects on your blood sugars.

• Working the overnight shift is usually not a great problem, especially if the weekend schedule does not vary greatly from the weekday schedule.

- If you work a rotating shift, it may be worthwhile staying on a single shift until the pump is correctly set. Talk with your employer to see if this can be done. If blood sugar control is poor and you work a rotating shift, seek the help of your physician/health care team to sort out this situation.

Carbohydrate Problems

One of the most critical elements for controlling blood sugars is to match carbohydrate intake to insulin doses. The most frequent cause for variable blood sugars is some problem related to the matchup between carbohydrates and the meal bolus. We'll discuss four areas in which problems with carbohydrates can occur. Again, a continuous monitor can assist you in pinning down what effect different carbs have on your readings and how the timing and size of the bolus balance these carbs. This allows a fast appraisal of the changes required for excellent control.

Measurement Errors

Good blood sugar control is difficult if you are not accurately measuring carbohydrates. When the amount of carbohydrate in a meal is unknown, it's impossible to give an accurate carbohydrate bolus. Problems can arise from inexperience in measuring carbohydrates, from frequently eating out where carbohydrate quantities are hard to estimate, or from simply not measuring.

Pattern:

If your basal rate tests are good but your blood sugars vary when you eat, consider that the problem may be in measuring carbohydrates. On your *Smart Charts*, look for a high or low blood sugar related to a particular meal, especially if the meal was eaten at a restaurant or friend's house, or if you haven't had this meal before.

Let's say you need 1 unit of Humalog for each 10 grams of carbohydrate. Suppose you usually eat 70 grams of carbohydrate for dinner and have great blood sugars with a 7-unit bolus, but one evening you have "70 grams" covered with a 7-unit bolus and your blood sugar rises. Be suspicious that you miscalculated the carbohydrate in that meal.

What To Do:

- If you suspect inaccurate measurement is a problem, review how to measure carbohydrates with your nutritionist or physician/health care team.

- If you eat out often, try eating a favorite meal at the same restaurant until you can cover it well with a bolus. On each occasion, record how many grams of carbohydrate you estimate the meal contains and how many units of insulin you took to cover it. It will become obvious after a few tries how many units you need for that meal. This carbohydrate bolus then will indicate to you the actual number of grams of carbohydrate in the meal. Some of the books listed in Chapter 7 are very handy for eating out. They give a comprehensive list of foods found in different types of restaurants and the number of grams of carbohydrate they contain.

• Take your gram scale and the Carb Factors in Appendix A with you to the restaurant. Weigh your food and calculate the grams of carbohydrate in it. Don't worry. People do strange things in restaurants. Pretend you are a government inspector or food critic. Some self-consciousness will be more than offset by your improved control and the extra service you receive from the waiter.

Variations in Meal Size and Timing

Although pumping is the best method for managing variety in your life, variations in the size and timing of meals still can make stable blood sugars hard to achieve, especially if your carbohydrate boluses have never been tested or the testing was inconsistent due to a free-form lifestyle.

Pattern:

Here the pattern is the lack of pattern, with only random day-to-day variation. This variation is easy to spot on your charts. Blood sugars will rise and fall, but more importantly the timing of meals and the carbohydrate in them will vary significantly from one day to the next.

What To Do:

Allow yourself the chance to stabilize. Eat meals with the same amount of carb in them and at the same time every day for a few weeks as you first go on your pump or if your blood sugar control has been poor. Avoid foods high in sugar or fat. Give yourself the opportunity to solve blood sugar problems by temporarily living life more routinely. Set your pump to match this consistency, and once you're well-controlled, begin reintroducing variety into your life. You'll find you can handle the changes you want much easier on the basis of stabilized blood sugars.

Variations in the Glycemic Index

As noted in Chapter 7, not all carbohydrates are equal. Fifty grams of carbohydrate from ice cream can have an effect on your blood sugar totally different from that of fifty grams from a bowl of Cornflakes®. Although you're eating the same amount of carbohydrate, you'll find that your blood sugar rises higher and faster when you have the Cornflakes®.

When nutritionists realized that different carbohydrates can affect blood sugars differently, they attempted to quantify these differences by developing a glycemic index. A single glycemic index that fits everyone's food response cannot be developed due to individual variations. A variety of glycemic indexes exists, each providing a rough guide to how different foods will affect your blood sugar. Table 7.5 on page 66 averages the glycemic index for a variety of carbohydrates from several studies done by David Jenkins and others.[86,87,88]

Pattern:

Foods high on the glycemic index will show up on your postmeal blood sugar readings. If you start with 82 mg/dl (4.6 mmol), shoot up to 317 mg/dl (17.6 mmol) two hours later, and are back down to 123 mg/dl (6.8 mmol) before the next meal, you have covered your carbohydrate with the correct bolus. However, you either did not take your insulin soon enough before the meal or you ate a carbohydrate with a high glycemic index.

What To Do:

• Refer to the Glycemic Index on page 74. Check the foods you are eating against those listed. If your foods have a high rating, switch to foods that have a lower rating.

• Avoid foods with a high glycemic rating. If you eat them, try taking your meal bolus earlier than usual to offset this faster acting carbohydrate.

• Shift to different types or brands of foods. Instead of a wheat or corn-based cereal, try one made from oats or rice, such as Cheerios®, or one with more fiber, such as All Bran® or Shredded Wheat and Bran®. Instead of a banana, try strawberries. Instead of white rice, try brown rice. The book **Glucose Revolution** tells how to shift a diet toward lower glycemic index foods.

Unusual Food Effects

Some foods have unexpected effects on the blood sugar. Candies sweetened with sorbitol may send blood sugars higher than expected. Peanuts and pretzels often raise blood sugars more than expected. Chinese foods and pizza are renowned for their ability to raise blood sugars.

Occasionally, an individual will have a unique response to a food. One pumper had frequent, high blood sugars that were unexplainable until she noticed that they always occurred several hours after meals containing two or more ounces of cheese. Research has shown that pizza raises blood sugars higher than the carbohydrate content suggests it should,[89] confirming the experience many people have had with it. Some have noted that pizza that is lower in fat, such as a vegetarian one, does not raise the blood sugar as high.

Pattern:

Look for a consistent rise in your blood sugar when you eat a particular food.

What To Do:

• Write down all the foods you eat on your charts, not just the carbohydrates.

• If you suspect a particular food affects your blood sugar, record your blood sugar readings when you eat it. Compare these readings to other meals with similar amounts of carbohydrate to see if there's a difference. If you are suspicious of a low carb food such as cheese or meat, leave it out or reduce its quantity to see what effect it is having. If you see a pattern of rising blood sugars after eating a suspected food, eliminate it from your meals or reduce the amount you eat.

• If you suspect blood sugar variability because of your foods, you may need the assistance of your physician or nutritionist to sort it out. Be sure to seek their advice if you suspect you have a food-related problem, but are unable to determine its source.

Stress

Stress is a natural part of being human. Without stress, we would not have the challenges that offer growth, the conflicts that pinpoint areas of our personality in need of change, nor the losses from which to gather strength. Nonetheless, stress can be overwhelming at times. Difficult times occur with an extended illness, the death of a family member or friend, or a problematic work situation or relationship. The combination of several factors may occur at one time.

Stress interferes with blood sugar control in several ways. When stressful events occur, it is difficult to continue normal patterns of living. Eating, sleeping and exercise all may be altered. Sleep may be lost during periods of stress, exercise and other calming activities may be put aside, and fast foods high in sugar and fat may be eaten more often. Difficulties in controlling blood sugars during stress are often related to the difficulty in maintaining a sense of order in daily life.

Stress also interferes with blood sugar control through an excessive release of stress hormones. Fight-or-flight hormones help us remain alert and active during stress. Unfortunately, they also interfere with insulin's action, and cause extra glucose to be produced and released into the blood. This results in higher blood sugars than usual and the need for more insulin.

Emotions and blood sugars are interrelated. During emotional periods, blood sugars usually rise. High blood sugars cause more stress hormones to be released, and these then magnify emotional reactions. Elevated blood sugars can also cause changes within brain cells that promote depression and irritability. The result is an impaired ability to deal with the stress at hand.

Stress and frustration can also result from the challenge of caring for your diabetes. As you are learning to control your blood sugar, frustration from the seeming magnitude of the job can set in. Ongoing attention to detail can be stressful or even boring, especially when results are slow to be seen.

Pattern:

Generally, little pattern exists except that your blood sugars will rise after a stressful event. Some stress, especially that related to work, may lessen on weekends or during vacations. If you feel like a totally different person when you have had a few days off or you find your blood sugars are much easier to control at these times, consider carefully how much stress you may be under. Others often see the extent of our stress before we do, and their comments may be the first indication of our own level of stress.

What To Do:

- Practice good eating habits all the time. If you avoid candy bars when life is going well, you are less likely to pick up a candy bar when stress hits.

- Test your blood sugars, and use a continuous monitor, if available, to track your control at all times. When stress occurs, testing and exercise are often the first things dropped from your lifestyle. Testing makes normal blood sugars possible, and with normal blood sugars, brain function improves and stress hormone levels are lower. Whatever the source of stress, it can be handled better when you are in good control.

- Take time daily to exercise, especially when stressed. A walk can do wonders. Exercise releases endorphins in the brain to help you feel better and handle stress better. It also makes the cells more sensitive to insulin so that control is easier.

- Be aware that the demands of blood glucose monitoring, counting carbohydrates, and blood glucose regulation can be overwhelming at times. Take a break from these routines for one or two days when you need one. Determine how much time off you need to clear your mind. Take the time needed, and come back to your monitoring with new vigor.

- If you feel frustrated by your blood sugar readings or doubt that you can make any sense out of your *Smart Charts,* seek the help of someone who does not share your frustration. Talk with your physician for help or for a referral to someone who specializes in blood sugar control.

- How you respond to stress is largely a learned process. If you note frequent high blood sugars following job pressure, arguments, or bad news, seek the advice of a specialist in how to better handle your responses. Stress management classes are offered by community colleges and by many employers.

- Talk. Stress is always worse when carried alone. Share your feelings, worries, guilt, and pain with others. No burden is too great to share with others and sharing real concerns can strengthen relationships.

Eloquence is logic on fire.

Lyman Beecher

Wrap Up

Learning to control blood sugars is individualized to each person's needs. The process involves learning more about who you are. In adding an insulin pump to your life, expect to encounter periods where you will meet new challenges. There is no way for you to master blood sugar control and pumping without learning from a few mistakes.

Blood sugar control is so challenging that problems with fine tuning are inevitable at times. Besides patience, it helps to have the assistance of a knowledgeable support team. Good control happens faster when you are guided by a full array of professionals.

You are responsible for collecting and recording the information related to your blood sugars, but a health professional's trained eyes can spot important details and patterns in your charts that you may miss. Their experience will help you deal with the questions and problems that arise. How quickly you succeed in your effort at control depends to a large extent on how well you use the knowledge and support of your physician/health care team.

Another helpful aid, if available in your community, is a support group. Support groups are attended by people who have diabetes, their relatives, friends, and local health professionals. They provide an opportunity for everyone to catch up on the latest news in diabetes and to help one another with advice and information. Members of support groups often help each other accept diabetes and deal with it more effectively. They understand the rewards and difficulties of having diabetes better than people outside the group who haven't shared your experiences.

If you have a support group available, join it for the friendship and information it provides. If none exists, consider forming one. You need no agenda, just the desire to know and share your experience with other people with diabetes.

We hope the information in this book helps you toward your goal. We learned a great deal in writing it. We tried to keep you, our reader, in mind as we wrote so that our concepts fit your needs and are clear and understandable to you.

We give our wholehearted support for your success as you use your insulin pump to improve your blood sugars and health. You've already come far, simply by engaging in this process. Our best to you on your adventure.

Counting Carbs With A Scale & Carb Factors

Few foods, other than table sugar and lollipops, are totally carbohydrate. The Carb Factors provided on the following pages give the amount of carbohydrate in 1 gram of that particular food. To find out how much carbohydrate you are eating in a particular food, do a simple calculation:

1. Weigh the food on a gram scale to get its total weight, or check the label to find the weight in grams.

2. Then find that food and its Carbohydrate Factor in one of the Food Groups listed below.

3. On a calculator, multiply the food's weight in grams by its Carbohydrate Factor.

4. The answer is the number of grams of carbohydrate you are eating.

Example: Let's say you place a small apple on a gram scale and find that it weighs 100 grams. You look up its Carb Factor and find that it is 0.13. You then multiply 100 grams by 0.13 to get the carbohydrate you will be eating:

100 grams of apple X .13 = 13 grams of carbohydrate

Additional Information

Carbohydrate Factors give the actual concentration of carbohydrate in foods. For instance, apples are 13% carbohydrate (most of their weight is water); raisins are 77% carbohydrate by weight, and bagels contain 56% carbohydrate by weight. Both apple juice and regular sodas are 12% carbohydrate, although the carbohydrate in apple juice is higher in fructose, while a regular soda has more of its carbohydrate as sucrose or sugar.

Cranberry juice is even richer in carbohydrate at 16%, while grapefruit juice contains only 9% by weight. A 6-oz. glass of cranberry juice will therefore contain almost twice as much carbohydrate as an identical glass of grapefruit juice. Because it contains more carbohydrate, the glass of cranberry juice can raise the blood sugar nearly twice as far as the same amount of grapefruit juice. It will also require almost twice as much insulin to cover it.

Carb Factors For Various Foods

Beverages		Cold Cereals, Dry		Desserts and Sweets	
carbonated soda	.12	All Bran™	.78	apple butter	.46
chocolate milk	.11	Cheerios™	.70	banana bread	.47
eggnog	.08	Corn Chex™	.89	brownie with nuts	.50
flavored instant coffee	.06	Corn Flakes™	.84	cakes: angel food	.60
milk	.04	Fruit and Fiber™	.78	coffee	.52
punch	.11	granola	.68	fruit	.57
Alcoholic Beverages		Grapenuts™	.83	sponge	.55
beer: regular	.04	NutriGrain™	.86	candies: caramel	.76
light	.02	Product 19™	.77	fudge with nuts	.69
champagne	.01	Puffed Wheat™	.77	hard	.96
liqueurs	.30	Raisin Bran™	.75	jelly beans	.93
wine: dry	.04	Shredded Wheat™	.81	lollipops	.99
sweet	.12	Special K™	.76	peanut brittle	.73
Breads and Grains		Rice Krispies™	.88	chocolate syrup	.65
bagel	.56	Total™	.79	cookies: animal	.80
barley, uncooked	.77	Wheaties™	.80	chocolate chip	.59
biscuits	.45	**Hot Cereals, Cooked**		fig bar	.71
bread	.53	corn grits	.11	gingersnap	.80
bread drumbs	.74	Cream of Wheat™	.14	oatmeal & raisin	.72
bread sticks	.75	Farina™	.11	danish pastries	.46
corn starch	.83	oatmeal	.10	doughnuts: cake	.52
English muffin	.51	Roman Meal™	.14	jelly filled	.46
French toast	.26	Wheatena™	.12	fruit turnovers	.26
lentils	.19	**Combination Dishes**		honey	.76
macaroni: plain	.23	beef stew	.06	ice cream: plain	.21
cheese	.20	burrito	.24	cone	.30
muffins	.45	chicken pie	.17	bar	.25
pancakes & waffles: dry mix	.70	chili with beans	.11	ice milk	.23
prepared	.44	chili, no beans	.06	jams	.70
rice, cooked	.24	coleslaw	.14	jellies	.70
rolls	.60	fish and chips	.18	pies: apple	.37
spaghetti: plain	.26	lasagna	.16	blueberry	.34
with sauce	.15	macaroni and cheese	.20	cherry	.38
toast	.70	pizza	.28	lemon meringue	.38
tortillas: corn	.42	potato salad	.13	pecan	.23
flour	.58	spaghetti with meat sauce	.15	pumpkin	.23
wheat flour	.76	tossed salad	.05	preserves	.70
		tuna casserole	.13	sherbert	.32

Fruits					
apple	.13	grapes: concord	.14	pineapple: fresh	.14
applesauce	.10	European	.17	canned in water	.10
apricots: fresh	.13	green, seedless	.14	canned in juice	.15
canned in water	.10	grapefruit	.10	plums, fresh	.18
canned in juice	.14	honeydew	.08	canned in water	.12
dried	.60	lemons	.09	prunes: dehydrated	.91
banana	.20	limes	.10	dried, cooked	.67
blackberries	.12	mangoes	.17	raisins	.77
cantalope	.08	nectarines	.17	rasberries, fresh	.14
cherries: fresh, sweet red	.16	oranges	.12	strawberries, fresh	.08
fresh, sour red	.14	papayas	.10	strawberries: frozen, sweet	.26
canned in water	.11	peaches: fresh	.10	tangerines	.12
maraschino	.29	canned in water	.08	watermelon	.06
cranberry sauce, sugar	.36	canned in juice	.12		
dates, dried and pitted	.67	pears: fresh	.15		
figs: fresh	.18	canned in water	.09		
dried	.62	persimmons: Japanese	.20		
fruit cocktail, in water	.10	native	.34		

Juices		Juices, cont.		Snack Foods	
apple cider	.14	papaya	.12	almonds	.19
apple juice	.12	pineapple: canned	.14	cashews	.26
apricot	.12	frozen	.13	corn chips	.57
apricot nectar	.15	prune	.19	crackers: graham	.73
cranberry	.16	tomato	.04	round	.67
grape: bottled	.16	V-8	.04	rye	.50
grape: frozen	.13	**Sandwiches**		saltines	.70
grapefruit: fresh	.09	BLT	.19	marshmallows	.78
canned	.07	chicken salad	.24	mixed nuts	.18
frozen	.09	club	.13	onion dip	.10
grapefruit-orange: canned	.10	egg salad	.22	peanut butter	.17
frozen	.11	hot dog with bun	.26	peanuts	.20
lemon	.08	peanut butter and jelly	.50	pecans	.20
lemonade, frozen	.11	tuna salad	.24	pistachios	.19
orange: fresh	.11			popcorn, popped, no butter	.78
canned, unsweet	.10			potato chips	.50
canned, sweet	.12			pretzels	.75
frozen	.11			sunflower seeds, no shell	.19
orange-apricot	.13			walnuts	.15

Vegetables

artichole	.10	carrots: raw	.10	peppers	.05
asparagus	.04	cooked	.07	potatoes: baked	.21
avacado	.05	cauliflower: raw	.05	boiled	.15
bamboo shoots	.05	cooked	.04	hash browns	.29
beans: raw green	.07	celery	.04	French fries	.34
cooked green	.05	chard, raw	.05	chips	.50
beans: kidney, lima, pinto,		corn: canned	.06	pumpkin	.08
red, white	.21	steamed, off cob	.19	radishes	.04
beans sprouts	.06	sweet, creamed	.20	sauerkraut	.04
beets, boiled	.07	cucumber	.03	spinach	.04
beet greens, cooked	.03	eggplant, cooked	.04	soybeans	.11
broccoli	.06	lettuce	.03	squash: summer, cooked	.03
brussel sprouts, cooked	.06	mushrooms	.04	winter, baked	.15
cabbage: raw	.05	okra	.05	winter, boiled	.09
cooked	.04	onions	.07	tomatoes	.05
Chinese, raw	.03	parsnips	.18	turnips	.05
Chinese, cooked	.01	peas	.12		

Dressings, Sauces, Condiments

bacon bits	.19	mustard	.04	pickle relish, sweet	.34
BBQ sauce	.13	olives	.04	soy sauce	.10
catsup	.25	pickles, sweet	.36	spaghetti sauce	.09
cheese sauce	.06	salad dressings: blue cheese	.07	steak sauce	.09
chili sauce	.24	ceasar	.04	sweet & sour sauce	.45
hollandaise sauce	.08	French	.17	tartar sauce	.04
horseradish	.10	Italian	.07	tomato paste	.19
mayonnaise	.02	Russian	.07	Worcestershire sauce	.18

References

[1] Pickup JC, White MC, Keen H, Parsons JA, and Alberti KG: Long-term continuous subcutaneous insulin infusion in diabetics at home. *Lancet* 2, 8148: 870-873, 1979.

[2] D. Fedele et. al.: Influence of continuous insulin infusion (CSII) treatment on diabetic somatic and autonomic neuropathy. *J Endocrinol Invest* 7: 623-628, 1984.

[3] A.J. Boulton, J. Drury, B. Clarke, and J.D. Ward: Continuous subcutaneous insulin infusion in the management of painful diabetic neuropathy. *Diabetes Care* 5: 386-390, 1982.

[4] G. Viberti: Correction of exercise-induced microalbuminuria in insulin-dependent diabetics after 3 weeks of subcutaneous insulin infusion. *Diabetes* 30: 818-823, 1981.

[5] K. Dahl-Jorgensen et al.: Effect of near normoglycemia for two years on progression of early diabetic retinopathy, nephropathy, and neuropathy: the Oslo study. *BMJ* 293: 1195-1201, 1986.

[6] T. Olsen et. al.: Diabetic retinopathy after 3 years' treatment with continuous subcutaneous insulin infusion. *Acta Ophthalmol* (Copenh) 65: 185-189, 1987.

[7] H.L. Eichner et. al.: Reduction of severe hypoglycemic events in Type I (insulin dependent) diabetic patients using continuous subcutaneous insulin infusion. *Diabetes Research* 8: 189-193, 1988.

[8] E. Chantelau, M. Spraul, I. Muhlhauser, et. al.: Long-term safety, efficacy and side-effects of continuous subcutaneous insulin infusion treatment for Type I (insulin-dependent) diabetes mellitus: a one center experience. *Diabetologia* 32: 421-426, 1989.

[9] H. Beck-Nielsen, B. Richelsen, C. Hasling, et. al.: Improved in vivo insulin effect during continuous subcutaneous insulin infusion in patients with IDDM. *Diabetes* 33: 832-837, 1984.

[10] A.O. Marcus: Patient selection for insulin pump therapy. *Practical Diabetology* (November, 1992) 12-18.

[11] C. Binder et al.: Insulin pharmacokinetics. *Diabetes Care* 7: 188-199, 1984.

[12] T. Lauritzen et al.: Pharmacokinetics of continuous subcutaneous insulin infusion. *Diabetologia* 24: 326-329, 1983.

[13] Guerci B, meyer L, Delbachian I, Kolopp M, Ziegler O, and Drouin P: Blood glucose control on Sunday in IDDM patients: intnesified conventional therapy versus contiuous insulin infusion. *Diabetes Res Clin Pract* 40: 175-180, 1998.

[14] I. Lager et. al.: Reversal of insulin resistance in Type I diabetes after treatment with continuous subcutaneous insulin infusion. *BMJ* 287: 1661-1663, 1983.

[15] Ohkubo Y, Kishikawa H, Araki E, et. al.: Intensive insulin therapy prevents the progression of diabetic microvascular complications in Japanese patients with non-insulin-dependent diabetes mellitus: a randomized prospective 6-year study. *Diabetes Res Clin Pract* 28: 103-117, 1995.

[16] Georgopoulos A, Margolis S, Bachorik P, and Kwiterovich PO: Effect of improved glycemic control on the response of plasma triglycerides to ingestion of a saturated fat load in normotriglyceridemic and hypertriglyceridemic diabetic subjects. *Metabolism* 37: 866-871, 1988.

[17] Valensi P, Moura I, Le Magoarou M, Paries J, Perret G, Attali JR: Short-term effects of continuous subcutaneous insulin infusion treatment on insulin secretion in non-insulin-dependent overweight patients with poor glycaemic control despite maximal oral anti-diabetic treatment. *Diabetes Metab* 23: 51-57, 1997.

[18] Ilkova H, Glaser B, Tunckale A, Bagriacik N, and Cerasi E: Induction of long-term glycemic control in newly diagnosed type 2 diabetic patients by transient intensive insulin treatment. *Diabetes Care* 20: 1353-1356, 1997.

[19] Pein et. al.: *Diabetologia*: 39, #847, 1996

[20] R.S. Mecklenburg et al.: Acute complications associated with insulin infusion pump therapy. *JAMA* 252: 3265-3269, 1984.

[21] J.J. Bending et al.: Complications of insulin infusion pump therapy. *JAMA* 253: 2644, 1985.

[22] R. Renner: Therapy of Type 1 diabetes with insulin pumps; *Diamet*, June, 1991.

[23] E. Van Ballegooie, J.M. Hooymans, Z. Timmerman, et. al.: Rapid deterioration of diabetic retinopathy during treatment with continuous subcutaneous insulin infusion. *Diabetes Care* 7:236-242, 1984.

[24] D. Dahl-Jorgensen, O. Brinchmann-Hansen, K.F. Hansen, et. al.: Transient deterioration of retinopathy when multiple insulin injection therapy and CSII is started in IDDM patients. *Diabetes* 33(1): 4A, 1984.

[25] LP Aiello, SE Bursell, A Clermont, E Duh, and GL King: Vascular endothelial growth factor-induced retinal permeability is mediated byprotein kinase C in vivo and suppressed by an orally effective beta-isoform-selective inhibitor. *Diabetes* 46: 1473-80, 1997.

[26] SE Bursell, C Takagi, et al.: Specific retinal diacylglycerol and protein kinase C beta isoform modulation mimics abnormal retinal hemodynamics in diabetic rats. *Invest Ophthalmol Vis Sci* 38: 2711-20, 1997.

[27] M Kunisaki, SE Bursell, F Umeda, H Nawata, and GL King: Prevention of diabetes-induced abnormal retinal blood flow by treatment with d-alpha-tocopherol. *Biofactors* 7: 55-67, 1998.

[28] M Lu, M Kuroki, S Amano, et al.: Advanced glycation end products increase retinal vascular endothelial growth factor expression. *J Clin Invest* 15: 1219-24, 1998.

[29] The Diabetes Control and Complications Trial Research Group: The effect of intensive treatment of diabetes on the development and progression of long-term complications in insulin-dependent diabetes mellitus. *N Engl J Med* 329: 977-986, 1993.

[30] Bode BW, Steed RD, and Davidson PC: Reduction in severe hypoglycemia with long-term continuous subcutaneous insulin infusion in type 1 diabetes. *Diabetes Care* 19: 324-327, 1996.

[31] I.B. Hirsch, R. Farkas-Hirsch and P.D. Cryer: Continuous subcutaneous insulin infusion for the treatment of diabetic patients with hypoglycemic unawareness. *Diabetes Nutr Metab* 4: 1-3, 1991.

[32] R. Farkas-Hirsch and I.B. Hirsch: Continuous subcutaneous insulin infusion (CSII): A review of the past and its implementation for the future. March/April, 1994 issue of *Diabetes Spectrum*.

[33] C.G. Fanelli, L. Epifano, A.M. Rambotti, S. Pampanelli, A. DiVincenzo, F. Modarelli et. al.: Meticulous prevention of hypoglycemia normalizes the glycemic thresholds and magnitude of most of neuroendocrine responses to, symptoms of, and cognitive function during hypoglycemia in intensively treated patients with short-term IDDM. *Diabetes* 42: 1683-1689, 1993.

[34] H.U. Janka, J.H. Warram, L.I. Rand and A.S. Krolewski: Risk factors for progression of background retinopathy in long-standing IDDM. *Diabetes* 38: 460-464, 1989.

[35] Ohkubo Y, Kishikawa H, Araki E, Miyata T, Isami S, Motoyoshi S, Kojima Y, Furuyoshi N, Shichiri M: Intensive insulin therapy prevents the progression of diabetic microvascular complications in Japanese patients with non-insulin-dependent diabetes mellitus: a randomized prospective 6-year study. *Diabetes Res Clin Pract* 1995 May;28(2):103-17

[36] K. Dahl-Jorgensen et al.: Reduction of urinary albumin excretion after 4 years of continuous insulin infusion in insulin-dependent diabetes mellitus. *NEJM* 316: 1376-1383, 1987.

[37] E. Chantelau, H Weiss, U. Weber, G.E. Sonnenberg, and M. Berger: Four-year followup of retinal status and glycosylated hemoglobin in patients with insulin-dependent diabetes mellitus. *Diabete & Metabolisme* 14: 259-263, 1988.

[38] Klein R and Klein BE: Relation of glycemic control to diabetic complications and health outcomes. *Diabetes Care* 1998 Dec;21 Suppl 3:C39-43

[39] V Melki, E Renard, V Lassmann-Vague, et al.: Improvement of HbA1c and blood glucose stability in IDDM patients treated with lispro insulin analog in external pumps. *Diabetes Care* 21(6): 977-82, 1998

[40] Renner R, Pfutzner A, Trautmann M, Harzer O, Sauter K, Landgraf R: Use of insulin lispro in continuous subcutaneous insulin infusion treatment. Results of a multicenter trial. German Humalog-CSII Study Group. *Diabetes Care* 22(5): 784-8, 1999

[41] Lougheed WD, Zinman B, Strack TR, Janis LJ, Weymouth AB, Bernstein EA, Korbas AM, Frank BH: Stability of insulin lispro in insulin infusion systems. *Diabetes Care* 20(7): 1061-5, 1997

[42] Zinman B, Tildesley H, Chiasson JL, Tsui E, Strack T: Insulin lispro in CSII: results of a double-blind crossover study. *Diabetes* 46(3): 440-3, 1997

[43] V.A. Koivisto and P. Felig: Alterations in insulin absorption and in blood glucose control associated with varying insulin injection sites in diabetic patients. *Ann Intern Med* 92: 59-61, 1980.

[44] J.P. Bantle et al.: Rotation of the anatomic regions used for insulin injections and day-to-day variability of plasma glucose in Type I diabetic subjects. *JAMA* 263: 1802-1806, 1990.

[45] M.H. Tanner et. al.: Toxic shock syndrome from staphylococcus areus infection at insulin pump infusion sites. *JAMA* 259: 394-395, 1988.

[46] A. Pietri and P. Raskin: Cutaneous complications of chronic continuous subcutaneous insulin infusion therapy. *Diabetes Care* 4: 624-627, 1981.

[47] J.S. Christiansen et. al.: Clinical outcome of using insulin at 40 IU/ml and 100 IU/ml in pump treatment. Results of a controlled multi-center trial. *Acta Med Scan* 221: 385-393, 1987.

[48] N. Perrotti, D. Santoro, S. Genovese et al.: Effect of digestible carbohydrates on glucose control in insulin-dependent diabetic patients. *Diabetes Care* 7: 354-359, 1984.

[49] G. Boden and F. Jadali: Effects of lipid on basal carbohydrate metabolism in normal men. *Diabetes* 40: 686-692, 1991.

[50] D.M. Mott, S. Lilloija, and C. Bogardus: Overnutrition induced decrease in insulin action for glucose storage: in vivo and in vitro in man. *Metabolism* 35: 160-165, 1986.

[51] J.A. Marshall, S. Hoag, S. Shetterly and R.F. Hamman: Dietary fat predicts conversion from impaired glucose tolerance to NIDDM. *Diabetes Care* 17: 50-56, 1994.

[52] E. Ferrannini, E.J. Barrett, S. Bevilacqua, R.A. DeFronzo: Effect of fatty acids on glucose production and utilization in man. *J Clin Invest* 1983; 72: 1737-1747.

[53] G.M. Reaven: Banting Lecture 1988: Role of insulin resistance in human disease. *Diabetes* 37: 1595-1607, 1988.

[54] P. Halfon, J. Belkhadir and G. Slama: Correlation between amount of carbohydrate in mixed meals and insulin delivery by artificial pancreas in seven IDDM subjects. *Diabetes Care* 12: 427-429, 1989.

[55] F.Q. Nuttall, A.D. Mooradian, M.C. Gannon et al.: Effect of protein ingestion on the glucose and insulin response to a standardized oral glucose load. *Diabetes Care* 7: 465-470, 1984.

[56] J. Beyer et. al.: Assessment of insulin needs in insulin-dependent diabetics and healthy volunteers under fasting conditions. *Horm Metab Res Suppl* 24: 71-77, 1990.

[57] W. Bruns et. al.: Nocturnal continuous subcutaneous insulin infusion: a therapeutic possibility in labile Type I diabetes under exceptional conditions. Z. *Gesamte Inn Med* 45: 154-158, 1990.

[58] K. Haakens et. al.: Early morning glycaemia and the metabolic consequences of delaying breakfast/morning insulin. A comparison of continuous subcutaneous insulin infusion and multiple injection therapy with human isophane or human Ultralente at bedtime. *Scand J Clin Lab Invest* 49: 653-659, 1989.

[59] G. Perriello, P. De Feo, E. Torlone, et. al.: The Dawn Phenomenon in Type I (insulin-dependent) diabetes mellitus; magnitude, frequency, variability, and dependency on glucose counterregulation and insulin sensitivity. *Diabetologia* 42: 21-28, 1991.

[60] P. Hildebrandt, K. Birch, B.M. Jensen, and C. Kuhl: Subcutaneous insulin infusion: Change in basal infusion rate has no immediate effect on insulin absorption rate. *Diabetes Care* 9: 561-564, 1986.

[61] I. Lager et. al.: Reversal of insulin resistance in Type I diabetes after treatment with continuous subcutaneous insulin infusion. *BMJ* 287: 1661-1663, 1983.

[62] H. Beck-Nielsen et. al.: Improved in vivo insulin effect during continuous subcutaneous insulin infusion in patients with IDDM. *Diabetes* 33: 832-837, 1984.

[63] H. Beck-Nielsen et. al.: Improved in vivo insulin effect during continuous subcutaneous insulin infusion in patients with IDDM. *Diabetes* 33: 832-837, 1984.

[64] J.M. Stephenson et al.: Dawn Phenomenon and Somogyi Effect in IDDM. *Diabetes Care* 12: 245-251, 1989.

[65] D. Cox, L. Gonder-Frederick, W. Polonsky, D. Schlundt, B. Kovatchev and W. Clark: Recent hypoglycemia influences the probability of subsequent hypoglycemia in Type I patients. Abstract 399, ADA Conference 1993.

[66] B. Zinman: The physiologic replacement of insulin. *NEJM* 321: 363-370, 1989.

[67] J. Walsh and R. Roberts: *Pumping Insulin*: Everything in a book for successful use of an insulin pump. (2nd ed.) Torrey Pines Press, San Diego, pgs. 68-71, 1994.

[68] SN Davis, S Fowler, and F Costa: Hypoglycemic Counterregulatory responses differ between men and women with Type 1 diabetes. *Diabetes* 49: 65-72, 2000.

[69] J. Anderson, S. Symanowski, and R. Brunelle: Safety of [Lys(B28), Pro(B29)] human insulin analog in long-term clinical trials. *Diabetes* 43(1): abstract 192, 1994.

[70] EA Boland, M Grey, A Oesterle, L Fredrickson, and WV Tamborlane: Continuous subcutaneous insulin infusion. A new way to lower risk of severe hypoglycemia, improve metabolic control, and enhance coping in adolescents with type 1 diabetes. *Diabetes Care* 22: 1779-84, 1999.

[71] A. Avogaro, P. Beltramello, L. Gnudi, A. Maran, A. Valerio, M. Miola, N. Marin, C. Crepaldi, L. Confortin, F. Costa, I. MacDonald and A. Tiengo: Alcohol intake impairs glucose counterregulation during acute insulin-induced hypoglycemia in IDDM patients. *Diabetes* 42: 1626-1634, 1993.

[72] T. Veneman, A. Mitrakou, M. Mokan, P. Cryer and J. Gerich: Induction of hypoglycemia unawareness by asymptomatic nocturnal hypoglycemia. *Diabetes* 42: 1233-1237, 1993.

[73] C.G. Fanelli, L. Epifano, A.M. Rambotti, S. Pampanelli, A. DiVincenzo, F. Modarelli, M. Lepore, B Annibale, M. Ciofetta, P. Bottini, F. Porcellati, L. Scionti, F. Santeusanio, P. Brunetti and G.B. Bolli: Meticulous prevention of hypoglycemia normalizes the glycemic thresholds and magnitude of most of neuroendocrine responses to, symptoms of, and cognitive function during hypoglycemia in intensively treated patients with short-term IDDM. *Diabetes* 42: 1683-1688, 1993.

[74] K. E. Powell et al.: Physical activity and chronic disease. *Am J Clin Nutr* 49: 999-1006, 1989.

[75] A. Festa, C.H. Schnack, A.D. Assie, P. Haber and G. Schernthaner: Abnormal pulmonary function in Type I diabetes is related to metabolic long-term control, but not to urinary albumin excretion rate. *Diabetes* 43 (1): abstract 610, 1994.

[76] J. Wahren: Glucose turnover during exercise in healthy man and in patients with Diabetes Mellitus. *Diabetes* 28(1): 82-88, 1979.

[77] P. Felig and J. Wahren: Role of insulin and glucagon in the regulation of hepatic glucose production during exercise. *Diabetes* 28(1): 71-75, 1979.

[78] P. White: Pregnancy complicating diabetes. *Am J Med* 7: 609-616, 1949.

[79] J. Pedersen: Fetal mortality in diabetics in relation to management during the latter part of pregnancy. *Acta Endocrinol* 15: 282-294, 1954

[80] J. Pedersen and E. Brandstrup: Fetal mortality in pregnant diabetics: strict control of diabetes with conservative obstetric management. *Lancet* I: 607a-612, 1956.

[81] J. Pedersen, L. Molsted-Pedersen and B. Andersen: Assessors of fetal perinatal mortality in diabetic pregnancy. *Diabetes* 23: 302-305, 1974.

[82] K. Fuhrmann, H. Reiher, K. Semmler, F. Fischer, M. Fisher and E. Glockner: Prevention of congenital malformations in infants of insulin-dependent diabetic mothers. *Diabetes Care* 6: 219-223, 1983.

[83] J.L. Kitzmiller, L.A. Gavin, G.D. Gin, L. Jovanovic-Peterson, E.K. Main and W.D. Zigrang: Preconception care of diabetes: Glycemic control prevents congenital anomalies. *JAMA* 265: 731-736, 1991.

[84] B. Rosenn, M. Miodovnik, C.A. Combs, J. Khoury and T.A. Siddiqi: Preconception management of insulin-dependent diabetes: Improvement of pregnancy outcome. *Obstet Gynecol* 77: 846-849, 1991.

[85] J.M. Steel, F.D. Johnstone, D.A. Hepburn and A. Smith: Can prepregnancy care of diabetic women reduce the risk of abnormal babies? *Br Med J* 301: 1070-1074, 1990.

[86] M. Miodovnik, C. Skillman, J.C. Holroyde, J.B. Butler, J.S. Wendel and T. A. Siddiqi: Elevated maternal glycohemoglobin in early pregnancy and spontaneous abortion among insulin-dependent diabetic women. *Am J Obstet Gynecol* 153: 439-442.

[87] J.L. Mills, J.L. Simpson, S.G. Driscoll, L. Jovanovic-Peterson, M. Van Allen, J.H. Aarons, B. Metzger, et.al.: The National Institute of Child Health and Human Development: Diabetes in Early Pregnancy Study: Incidence of spontaneous abortion among normal women and insulin-dependent diabetic women whose pregnancies were identified within 21 days of conception. *NEJM* 319: 1617-1623, 1988.

no 83

[88] L. Jovanovic-Peterson, M. Druzin and C.M. Peterson: Effect of euglycemia on the outcome of pregnancy in insulin-dependent diabetic women as compared with normal control subjects. *Am J Med* 71: 921-927, 1981.

[89] C.A. Combs, B. Wheeler, E. Gunderson, L. Gavin, and J.L. Kitsmiller: Significance of microproteinuria in the first trimester of pregnancies complicated by diabetes. *Diabetes* 39: 36A, 1990.

[90] D.J.A. Jenkins, T.M.S. Wolever and A.L. Jenkins: Starchy foods and glycemic index. *Diabetes Care* 11: 149-59, 1988.

[91] D.J.A. Jenkins, T.M.S. Wolever, et al.: Glycemic index of foods: a physiologic basis for carbohydrate exchange. *Amer J Clin Nutr* 34: 362-66, 1981.

[92] T.M.S. Wolever, L Katzman-Relle et al.: Glycemic index of 102 complex carbohydrate foods in patients with diabetes. *Nutr Res* 14: 651-69, 1994.

[93] J.A. Ahern, P.M. Gatcomb, N.A. Held, W.A. Petit, W.V. Tamborlane: Exaggerated hyperglycemia after pizza meal in well-controlled diabetes. *Diabetes Care* 16: 578-580, 1993.

Glossary

Albuminuria

A condition in which high levels of a protein called albumin are found in the urine. Excess albumin in the urine is often a sign of early kidney disease.

Adult diabetes

Now called Type 2 or NIDDM (non-insulin dependent diabetes).

Basal Insulin or Rate

A continuous 24-hour delivery of insulin that matches background insulin need. When the basal rate is correctly set, the blood sugar does not rise or fall during periods in which the pump user is not eating. Basal rates are given as units/hour with typical rates between 0.4 u/hr and 1.6 u/hr for many pumpers.

Bolus

See Carb Bolus or High Blood Sugar Bolus.

Beta cells (b-cells)

Cells that make insulin and are found in the Islets of Langerhans within the pancreas.

Blood glucose level

The concentration of glucose in the blood (blood sugar). It is measured in milligrams per deciliter (mg/dl) in the U.S. or in millimoles (mmol) in other countries.

Body mass index (BMI)

A unit of measurement (kg/m^2) that describes weight in relation to height for people 20 to 65 years old.

Brittle diabetes

A so-called type of Type I diabetes in which the blood glucose level fluctuates widely from high to low, usually as a result of insulin doses not matching lifestyle factors. It often can be improved through a good treatment program, such as flexible insulin therapy or insulin pump therapy.

Carbohydrate

One of the three main constituents (carbohydrates, fats, and proteins) of foods. Carbohydrates (four calories per gram) are composed mainly of sugars and starches.

Carb Bolus

A spurt of insulin delivered quickly to match carbohydrates in an upcoming meal or snack. Most pumpers use between 1 unit of Humalog for each 5 grams of carbohydrate and 1 unit of Humalog for each 25 grams.

Carb counting

Counting the grams of carbohydrate in any food eaten. This is an effective way to determine the amount of insulin needed to maintain a normal blood sugar.

Catheter

The plastic tube through which insulin is delivered between the pump and the insertion set.

C-peptide

A byproduct of insulin production. Plasma C-peptide has a longer half-life than insulin and often is used to measure how much insulin a person is able to make. Generally, a level below 0.3 is defined as Type I diabetes.

CSII

Continuous subcutaneous insulin infusion, a fancy name for using an insulin pump.

DCCT

Diabetes Control and Complications Trial. The DCCT was a 9-year study of more than 1,400 people with Type 1 diabetes. Sponsored by the National Institute of Health, it showed that tight blood sugar control significantly reduces the risk of diabetic retinopathy, neuropathy, and nephropathy.

Dawn Phenomenon

An early morning rise in blood glucose levels, caused largely by the normal release of growth hormone that blocks insulin's effect during the early morning hours. It is more likely to raise blood sugar in Type I than Type II diabetes.

Diabetic coma

Loss of consciousness due to very high blood sugars. (See ketoacidosis)

Diabetic nephropathy

Kidney disease resulting from diabetes that usually has been poorly controlled for several years. There rarely are symptoms until very late in the disease.

Diabetic neuropathy

Damage to the nervous system most often resulting from poor control. Three different forms of neuropathy can be distinguished: peripheral neuropathy, sensory neuropathy, and autonomic neuropathy. Peripheral neuropathy affects the motor nerves, which can lead to problems with muscle movement and size. Sensory neuropathy impairs the nerves that control touch, sight, and pain perception. Autonomic neuropathy affects the nerves involved in such involuntary functions as digestion. Symptoms such as pain, loss of sensation, loss of reflexes, and/or weakness may occur.

Diabetic retinopathy

Damaged small blood vessels in the eye that can cause vision problems, including blindness.

Endogenous insulin

Insulin production within a person in the beta cells.

Exchange lists

Food within any particular list—starch/bread, meat, vegetable, fruit, milk, and fat—may be exchanged with other foods on the same list without changing the nutritional content of the diet.

Fasting plasma glucose (FPG) test

The test is taken after fasting for 8 to 10 hours, typically overnight. FPG level less than 110 mg/dL is normal; one between 110 and 126 mg/dL indicates impaired glucose tolerance, and one greater than 126 mg/dL supports a provisional diagnosis of diabetes.

Exchange

A serving of food that contains known and relatively constant amounts of carbohydrate, fat, and/or protein. The food is listed in an exchange by portion size determined by weight or measurement. There are exchanges for milk, fruit, meat, fat, bread, and vegetables.

Exogenous insulin

Insulin given by injection or pump; vital for Type 1 diabetes and needed by many with Type 2 diabetes.

Fat

One of the three main constituents (carbohydrate, fats, and protein) of foods. Fats occur alone as liquids or solids, such as oils and margarines, or they may be a component of other foods. Fats may be of animal or vegetable origin. They have a higher energy content than any other food (9 calories per gram).

Flexible insulin therapy (FIT)

Therapy that uses predetermined blood sugar targets and HBA1c values as goals. The therapy includes frequent blood sugar testing (at least four times a day). Carbohydrate content of food eaten, exercise, stress, and other factors are evaluated to determine insulin need. In early Type 2, no insulin or one to two injections may be needed. In later stages of Type 2 and in Type 1, insulin is delivered by three or more injections a day or by use of an insulin pump.

Gestational diabetes

Elevated blood sugars usually diagnosed during the last half of pregnancy and triggered by insulin resistance. Gestational diabetes increases the risk of perinatal mortality and the development of diabetes in the mother years following the pregnancy.

Glucagon

A hormone made by the pancreas that raises blood sugar levels. It is injected during severe low blood sugars to raise the blood sugar quickly by releasing glucose stored in the liver.

Glucose

A simple sugar, also known as dextrose, that is found in the blood and is used by the body for energy.

Glycogen

Glycogen is the form in which the liver and muscles store glucose. It may be broken down to active blood glucose during an insulin reaction, a fast, or exercise.

Glycosylated hemoglobin

Glycosylated hemoglobin levels reflect blood glucose during the previous two to three months. HbA1c is a form of glycosylated hemoglobin commonly used to assess blood glucose control in people with diabetes. Normal HbA1c levels are generally 4% to 6%. Diabetes treatment typically aims for a target HbA1c of less than 7%.

Gram

A small unit of weight in the metric system. Used in weighing food. One pound equals 453 grams.

High Blood Sugar Bolus

A spurt of insulin delivered quickly to bring a high blood sugar back to normal. For most pumpers, one unit will lower the blood sugar between 20 and 100 mg/dl or points (between 1 and 6 mmol).

Hormone

A chemical substance produced by a gland or tissue and carried by the blood to other tissues or organs, where it stimulates action and causes a specific effect. Insulin and glucagon are hormones.

Hyperglycemia

A higher than normal level of glucose in the blood (high blood sugar). Fasting serum glucose levels greater than 105 mg/dl (5.8 mmol) are suspect; greater than 126 mg/dl (7.0 mmol) are diagnostic. Acute symptoms include frequent urination, increased thirst, and weight loss. If left untreated, hyperglycemia results in chronic diabetes complications: cardiovascular disease, neuropathy, retinopathy, and nephropathy.

Hypertension

High blood pressure (excess blood pressure in the blood vessels). Found to aggravate diabetes and diabetic complications.

Hypoglycemia

A lower than normal level of glucose in the blood (low blood sugar), usually less than 60 mg/dl (3.3 mmol). Symptoms vary from confusion, nervousness, sweating, shakiness, headaches, and drowsiness to moodiness, or numbness in the arms and hands. If left untreated, severe hypoglycemia can cause loss of consciousness or convulsions.

Infusion Set

Refers to the hub, catheter, and insertion set.

Insertion Set

The part of the infusion set inserted through the skin. It may be a fine metal needle or a larger metal needle, which is removed to leave a small teflon catheter under the skin.

Insulin

A hormone secreted by the beta cells of the Islets of Langerhans in the pancreas. Needed by many cells to use glucose for energy.

IDDM

Insulin-dependent diabetes mellitus, now more commonly called Type 1 diabetes. This type of diabetes requires treatment with exogenous insulin. See also Type 1 diabetes.

Insulin reaction

A condition caused by a low blood sugar, usually caused, in turn, by too much insulin or too little food. Extra exercise, without a corresponding increase in food or decrease in insulin, also can be a cause. See symptoms under Hypoglycemia.

Insulin pump

A small, computerized, programmable device about the size of a beeper that can be programmed to send a continuous stream of insulin into the bloodstream as basal insulin, as well as larger amounts prior to meals as boluses. It replaces insulin injections. A pump delivers fast-acting insulin via a plastic catheter to either a teflon infusion set or a small metal needle inserted through the skin for gradual absorption into the bloodstream. Doses as small as 0.1 unit or less can be delivered with accuracy.

Insulin resistance

A basic metabolic abnormality underlying Type 2 diabetes. Insulin resistance describes reduced insulin sensitivity of cells to the action of insulin.

Interstitial fluid

A relatively clear fluid between cells in which glucose measurements can be made without drawing blood by puncturing a blood vessel.

Islets of Langerhans

Special groups of pancreatic cells that produce insulin and glucagon.

Ketoacidosis

A very serious condition in which the body does not have enough insulin. An excess release of free fatty acids causes high levels of ketones in the blood and urine. This acidic state takes hours or days to develop, with symptoms of abdominal pain, nausea, and vomiting. It also causes dehydration, electrolyte imbalance, rapid breathing, coma, and possibly death.

Ketones

Acidic byproducts of fat metabolism.

Nephropathy

See Diabetic nephropathy

Neuropathy

See Diabetic neuropathy

NIDDM

Non-insulin-dependent diabetes mellitus, or Type 2 diabetes. This type of diabetes may or may not require treatment with exogenous insulin. See also Type 2 diabetes.

Oral glucose tolerance test (OGTT)

A 2 or 3-hour test of plasma glucose with values over 200 mg/dL (> 11.1 mmol/L) used to confirm a suspected diagnosis of diabetes.

Pancreas

A gland positioned near the stomach that secretes insulin, glucagon, and many digestive enzymes.

Protein

One of the three main constituents (carbohydrate, fat, and protein) of foods. Proteins are made up of amino acids and are found in foods such as milk, meat, fish, and eggs. Proteins are essential constituents of all living cells and form important structures and enzymes. Proteins (four calories per gram) are burned at a slower rate than fats or carbohydrates.

Proteinuria

Protein in the urine. This may be a sign of kidney damage.

Reservoir/Syringe/Cartridge

A container which holds the fast-acting insulin inside a pump.

Retina

A very thin light-sensitive layer of nerves and blood vessels at the back of the inner surface of the eyeball.

Type 1 diabetes

Insulin-dependent diabetes mellitus (IDDM). In Type 1 diabetes the pancreas makes little or no insulin because the insulin-producing beta cells have been destroyed. This type of diabetes usually appears suddenly and most commonly in people younger than 30. Treatment consists of daily insulin injections or use of an insulin pump, a planned diet, regular exercise, and daily self-monitoring of blood glucose.

Type 2 diabetes

Non-insulin-dependent diabetes mellitus (NIDDM). Type 2 diabetes is associated with insulin resistance and impaired beta cell function. It sometimes is controlled by diet, exercise, and daily monitoring of glucose levels, but at other times oral antihyperglycemic agents or insulin injections are needed. Type 2 diabetes accounts for 90% to 95% of diabetes cases.

List Of Essential Phone Numbers:

My Doctor: _____ at ( ) _____-_____

My Nurse/educator: _____ at ( ) _____-_____

Pump representative: _____ at ( ) _____-_____

Pump company: _____ at ( ) _____-_____

School Care Plan For An Insulin Pump

Re: _____   Date: _____/_____/_____

To Whom It May Concern:

_____ is a patient in our Center with Type 1 Diabetes Mellitus (Insulin Dependent Diabetes Mellitus). To better control his/her diabetes, he/she is using insulin pump therapy.

An insulin pump is simply another way to deliver insulin. Through the pump, _____ receives insulin around the clock via a small needle or plastic tube which is inserted in his/her abdomen. _____ has been taught how to program the pump to deliver insulin, as he/she needs it. This means he/she will program the pump before each meal to give insulin in a dose determined by his/her fingerstick blood glucose test.

To take care of his/her diabetes at school, _____ will need to have the following items with him/her:

    — The insulin infusion pump, which is worn
    — Backup pump supplies (syringes, tubing, insulin), and regular syringe
    — Glucagon injection kit for severe low blood sugar
    — Blood glucose testing supplies (meter, strips, lancet device, and lancets)
    — Snack foods and water (to handle extremes of blood glucose)
    — Ketostix (to test urine ketones as needed)
    — _____

There may be times when _____ will need to be excused to test his/her blood sugar or ketones, or to use the bathroom. In case of a low blood sugar emergency, the pump can be stopped, although it is usually more important to raise the blood sugar with a drink or food that contains sugar. _____ can show you how to do this. If a severe low blood sugar should occur, the needle or catheter can easily be temporaily disconnected near the skin site, or completely untaped and removed from the skin (reattachment is essential within 30 to 60 minutes).

Pump therapy is a safe and effective way to manage diabetes. We are confident that _____ can handle this tool properly.

If you need further information, please contact his/her family or our office.

Sincerely,

_____

Index

Order Form for Pumping Insulin

Please send me _____ copies of Pumping Insulin at $23.95 each. I understand that I may return any books for a full refund within 30 days for any reason. (California residents add 7.75% sales tax ($1.86) for a cost of $25.81, plus shipping.) Call for discounts on quantity orders.

Name _____

Addr _____

City _____ State _____ Zip _____

Phone (____) _____ - _____

_____ copies of **Pumping Insulin** at $23.95 each (or $25.81 in California)

_____ *My Other CheckBooks* (includes *Pocket Pancreas* & 4 mos. *Smart Charts*) at $12.95

_____ *Smart Charts* (refill for 4 mos.) at $8.95

Shipping: $_____ ❑ Priority Mail $4 ❑ Bookrate $3 (Plus $1 for each add item)

Total $_____

Payment: ❑ Check
❑ Visa ❑ Mastercard ❑ American Express

cc #: _____ Exp. Date: _____/_____/_____

Signature: _____

Mail your order to: **Torrey Pines Press**
1030 West Upas St.
San Diego, CA 92103

Or call: (800) 988-4772
Or call or fax: (619) 497-0900